increase

the university of georgia press   athens & london

lia purpura) *increase*

Published by the University of Georgia Press
Athens, Georgia 30602
© 2000 by Lia Purpura
All rights reserved
Designed by Erin Kirk New
Set in 10.5 on 15 Minion
Printed and bound by Maple-Vail Book Group
The paper in this book meets the guidelines for
permanence and durability of the Committee on
Production Guidelines for Book Longevity of the
Council on Library Resources.

Printed in the United States of America
04   03   02   01   00   C   5   4   3   2   1

Library of Congress Cataloging-in-Publication Data
Purpura, Lia, 1964–
Increase / Lia Purpura.
p. cm.
ISBN 0-8203-2232-6 (alk. paper)
1. Pregnant women—United States—Biography.
2. Mothers—United States—Biography. 3. Pregnancy.
4. Childbirth. I. Title.
RG526 .P87 2000
618.2´0092—dc21
[B]   99-044066

British Library Cataloging-in-Publication Data available

for joseph

acknowledgments

I would like to thank:

My husband, Jed Gaylin, who encouraged endlessly and passionately, and who built in himself, in all ways, a home for us.

My mother and father, Maddalena and John Purpura, and my mother- and father-in-law, Rita and Ned Gaylin, who so willingly gave the gift of time.

A. V. Christie, Jane Satterfield, and Patricia Debney Watkins, mothers and writers—inspirations, all—for keen eyes, for sound thinking, and for making, out of thin, often frayed air, time to help.

Judith Kitchen, whose attentive care and light, insightful hand went above and beyond.

Carl Klaus, for the clear and generous lens focused on this work as it developed.

Josefina Sanchez-Calzada and Cindy Hollister—constant sources of calm, good wisdom.

Annabelle Cummings, for peace of mind—I couldn't have worked without it.

I am grateful to the MacDowell Colony and to the Center for Humanities at Loyola College in Maryland for supporting my work.

Excerpts from *Increase* have been published in *American Voice* and the *Georgia Review*.

increase

A blue X slowly crosses itself, first one arm, then the other in the small white window of the test. The blue is a wisp, a shading, a smoke, then a sketch when it ciphers a certainty. Blue crosscurrents of veins under skin; translucent, stalactite blue in the cave I'm becoming from this moment on. Robin's egg and the gaping mouths of baby birds. Blue in the face. Tributaries, from far away. Blue houses on china, and the curled lip of a near wave. Blue moons waxing inside, in time. I go downstairs to my husband and our friends, visiting from England with their new baby, and say "I'm pregnant" in the middle of their conversation.

X, the unknown, variable quantity. A kiss in a letter. Marked so when the name is as yet undetermined. Or cannot be spoken. Cannot be written.
A sign between figures, indicating dimension. Its speck of a heart. To find yourself here.

Pregnant *has a discernible heft as I drop it; it rings out, it is rung by the swift force of the moment. Which I stand under, as a child does, in a state of sought response*—what will they say?—*as a child presents a picture with flourish, as if on a platter, as if for a feast:* Here, see what I've done. Tell me, now, who I am.

We visited the cabin just for the day. After dinner I walked
down to the lake and sat on the prow of an overturned boat,
watching the bluegills float and dart, each with a dab of black
on its head. I sat like anyone deeply absorbed, without thought
to time, in the small necessity of the moment. I threw a piece
of bread I found and they lunged at it; they were so close,
within a foot of the shore, the dry sand, wholly alert and ready
to spring on anything good that came their way. The slightest
sweep of their fins kept them moving, and they drifted past
one another, not communicating—at least not in the silent
and complex way ants do, with a head-on transmission of
scent or passing glances. It seemed they would gather together
at intervals, but soon I saw their massing and recombining was
random, defined only by the instant, an angle of sun, a stirring
above them.

The small butterfly glowed with such cornflower urgency
that I needed to see it up close. And when it allowed that,
stopping at an algae-covered twig and folding up its radiant
wings to one small leaf, it was the color of sand darkened by
water; it was a perfect indentation hidden in itself, a hovering
thumbprint.

In the cabin on a small round table is a vase whose handle is
eye-level when I sit, reading beside it. A mark is visible where

the potter attached the handle, a long, glazed smudge in white with blue, etched petals spiraling up it. Rough swatches where the thing was turned can be seen just under the skin of blue wash: as the gesture pulled down, the neck was brought forth and a lip was formed. It is the motion of birth, any birth— rapid hands and a bloom emerging.

I dropped the smallest frog I could find into the cloud of fish. And the cloud moved upon the surface of the water. I did it to see the hungry flash converge. I wanted to see drive, instinct, and plunder; gifts snatched from the literal hand of . . . I wanted to see the fish turn to rays, their impulse struck from them, as a bell's music is struck from a silent core. And what was I now—bountiful as any god with a pile of thunder-bolts ready to hurl, all desire, all terrible abundance?

)))

To feel *ache* as the shape of a child moving, this early on, takes conjuring. It is a choice not unlike any choice of attention I might make in the course of a day, and one which depends, as so much does, on whim: I stop to touch the rough glaze on a cup. Anxious for assurance that all's well, vital, and muscularly fit, I can go for days without having to know this as physical certainty. And holding off knowing, I am cast back: I am that girl who watched a friend's older sister line her eyes in black and add bright blue, garish and creamy against her perfect face, getting ready to meet a boy at the park. And I think, *I don't have to do that yet.* I head back out into the open air, to the park across the street, to the pond and hills with my friend, who is smaller and faster than I am, who is already wearing, when she can steal it, a dab of her sister's best perfume.

)))

This clock, my body, changes daily, sweeps and hurtles forth, always forth. How well trained I've been all these years, to record its smallest quiet fluctuations: now a twinge, now a cramp, that's more a pressure, and that, a burning. In the doctor's office, walking to school, I begin to use the language of a tribe, not the private notations of flux and shift, not a brief registering of passing sensation. I say for the first time, about time, and to mark it—*trimester*.

july 14

Two nights ago we heard a rustling up from the sewer. There's a wide gap between the curb and the drain, and just below the grating, a pronounced ledge where a good-sized dog could fit (as happened three winters ago—one slipped in and sat shivering until a man with thick gloves from animal control pulled it out, a black lab, angry with fear.) One of the raccoons that lives there emerged. It walked in that mincing, menacing way on its small feet, pacing and loping in front of the sewer, mounting the curb, crossing the street and crossing again, back and forth like a leopard in a cage; but it was the noise it made that first drew us outside—a strange chuckling and hissing admixture, like a large bird's throaty click and then a higher-pitched warm-blooded quaver. Jed thought it might be rabid, and that seemed entirely possible—it wasn't yet dark outside, and the raccoon didn't flinch at the dogs barking nearby. But I knew, I was certain, that others were down there, or had been, and something was wrong. I knew that nothing could be more wrong than a young one missing. That this was a mother pacing and grieving. There could be no match for the fear, for the rage, which brought her out into the light, beside herself with remorse, which looks, I could see now, everything like craziness or disease.

july 18

The heavy brown, dark brown, orange-and-white cat walks along the cement path under the hanging vines and sits at the top of the stone steps. Here on its morning visit, it regards the tangle of green before reaching down to lick its paws and wash its ears and face. I've watched this cat for weeks, and it never once cocked its head the way a dog might, listening hard or in earnest surprise. It settles in. And sits. People on their porches do this, look lazily, privately out. I'd always assumed they were waiting for something to happen, or for something to come to them, bearing news. But their very posture precludes the gestures of surprise—jumping up, startling, rising from their chairs, angled toward the spectacle. They're in a kind of slow haze; yellow and fine-milled, it hangs in the heat around them. Of course, the porch-sitters might be quietly preparing—days, meals, trips, plots, stories, the next move—but the body's least conscious gestures are so often the mind's that it's hard to imagine even a moment's skittering behind such mute, immobile faces.

Late afternoons, though, the tiny cream-colored rabbit pours itself like raw silk down the hill out back, stopping to eat a ragged dandelion which it pulls into its mouth, without using its paws. Then a hollow stalk of chive. Then it goes, looking about, hopping to the next leaf and the next, eating, then nibbling, then trampling, tamping underfoot the whole range of green on its way somewhere, and somewhere else again.

july 19

A poem takes months or years to complete, to feel finished with, or to abandon entirely. Let's say from three to eighteen months. In that range of gestations, a poem can embody the way of the field mouse (23 days) and the way of the killer whale (517 days.) *Gestation* as time taking what it needs to complete the loop of a head, the loop of an arm, the loopy diversions in the nephrons of the kidney. A loop of thought: I have in me a way of time-marking, with all its attendant fears and burgeonings. "This poem is going nowhere" until suddenly, one day—which is not one day but an accumulation of, say, 217—it pops or floods, is closer than it's been before.

Basho: "A poet doesn't make a poem, something in the person naturally becomes a poem."

This waiting and working steadily is something I know, my body knows, I remind myself. I do not know it easily, but it is familiar—though it is true, too, that the familiar is passed over as quickly as pungent oddities are dismissed if not attended: *Why* we love whom and what we love. Remind and remember: because she cleans the table in brisk, perfectly efficient swipes. Because the tiger lily's throat is soaked with rust. His hands stir music into air. The mountain laurel's blooms begin as tight, webbed stars.

The child, then, as daily vow.

So if long growth is not only a constituting but also a renewing force—what, then, is *not* birth? The folding of darkness into light is a birth at every shaded increment. The relentless spring summer eases away, blows open, pays again into the fist of cold and the fist gradually loosened, worked flat again, until there, uncovered in the center of the palm, is the damp little tributary of sweat.

Which rises away.

july 26

I cannot think to work; nothing comes to me from the larger world; my throat is not catching around any sound at all. I sip water and swallow: just a powerful peristaltic squeeze and the pull and suck of distraction. I am here, but not filled by presence, not observed or taken away. I walk a closed shape and cannot get lost. Too rooted, I am a biological pulsing; though whatever keeps receptivity at bay is, at least, palpable. It is a thick mist of heavy air, a vertigo of stillness, and for this I find myself oddly thankful. I am stuck at work in a narrow hall, dull space between here and there while the home my body has become is busy furnishing away, rounding new corner after corner.

july 27

Early morning, and the neighborhood machines pare down
the green silence. Soon the hum of cicadas will crest over, and
each voice of the neighbor's three dogs will be distinct for a
moment. The whine of the saw will come closer, and the lower-
pitched mower start up, as, just now, two small planes sketch
and crosshatch the air more densely still.

The young rabbit is back; it is growing into its long legs,
losing the stiffness in them; the neck is thickening and fur
coarsening. And though more graceful than just weeks ago,
quick leaps more precise and measured, it is less like mercury
down the steps, has lost some of that liquid response to its own
uncontrolled speed. Alongside, squirrels run on raw nerve,
chatter and dig, trip and run circles around each other, at once
playful, aggressive, clever.

It is a morning of simultaneities, the time of day most like,
I imagine, motherhood—all cooking while thinking, bathing,
dressing while thinking, feeding and jotting, and always,
always anticipating need.

And what of the soft, meditative, and singular, not flying
from tree to tree in a tumult? What of its drive not to lift a
hand to shape or urge or temper anything at all? Not fixing or
feeding, tooling or tending, but sitting or standing by a
window, in a doorway, an eye, an ear for the day piling, as
plates, as cold food, papers, mail do, inexorably up.

By the time the big saw cuts out, it is already afternoon;
quiet sucks at the trees, as if a pressure applied has been
released, and the silence staggers around a bit until it's steady

again, upright, and can spread itself into the empty space, like blood cleanly welling after a quick cut.

august 1

For the past week or so I've been watching the Olympic sprinters, their granite faces and taut skin shaken loose by their great pounding strides. Even the ones who tire and crash and bleed make it seem natural to pick up and go on. The force each event exerts on the body and the single-mindedness with which the athletes approach their given tasks, grimly fierce or confident, seem both pure and absurd. I hear how the body can be trained to recover and keep going if the constant of pain is pushed through, worked with: one learns to become a harness, to keep the body both reined and in motion. More interesting, though, than these displays of control, which might even be taken for courage, has been the humility of the weightlifters. Many of them, after trying and failing to hoist record-breaking weights, dropped the black barbell to the floor, where it bounced menacingly a few times like a piston in a steelworks coming to a halt—and then laid their hands on the weights before walking away. It could have been a caress or a blessing. They'd simply shake their heads *no*, an open admission that the body could not pass that furthest point, that a limit had been reached and respected. No grumbling, no gnashing of teeth, no kicking the floor on which the weights fell—no anger at all toward the mute weights, those iron wheels hoisted and clamped in place with little pins.

The humility or the calm came, I imagine, from a full understanding of a bounded physical self, of what is possible and
likely, and ultimately, from undeniable proof of the body's
resistance. Here, too, was a wisdom, a practiced ability to
discern and accept the limits of one's body. And in that
acceptance one cannot be more simultaneously alone with and
accompanied by the body, refusing, then accepting its decrees.
I would like to think of pregnancy, then, not as a kind of
Olympics, with its language of heroics—of conqueror and
vanquished, of competitors surpassed or the underdog
miracle—but rather as a series of improvised moments,
beginning with a step onto a well-tended field, upon which the
drama of endurance will be played out.

august 4

By necessity, out of sheer survival and the logic of ages, the
powerless study the habits of the powerful—and so I must
learn, more adequately, the nature of pain, and how, with
intent, it comes on. I must learn of its whims and turnings, in
order to adapt to or measure myself against it. The myth of the
all-giving nature of motherhood, that *effacement*, may trace its
origin to the event of labor, where the body is first wracked,
and then, just hours hence, the pain has already drained from
clear memory, one act of erasure followed by another. Perhaps
the myth begins before this, with the actual language ascribed
to the earliest moments of labor: *effacement*, that act of the
cervix ripening into readiness: we do not say a *clarifying* of the

membrane; it is not a *translucence*, nor does it *shadow* or *sheer* or *unveil*. *Effacement*: already the language of diminishment locates the body as a site of loss. Loss amidst gain and the promise of riches, yes. But in the best cases I imagine "giving" birth not as a giving up or into, but a parceling out, a lucid weighing and judging of the body's readiness to meet and endure, or otherwise counter the fabled pain. I imagine it's something we've always been training for, with each reaction to pain's twinges or onslaughts, each recognition of our temperament and the accommodations we make for that temperament. If this is the case, and the threshold for pain is, for each of us, as a step up or down into a dwelling, then why, just yesterday, when a friend told of his wife's request for an epidural early in labor, did I feel a kind of judgment wash over? Why, nearly wordlessly, did I think "So, she couldn't do it herself," as if the cries of a hurt animal were not meant as a warning, not meant to call others like it close for help and for comfort.

august 8

Sharing. Shares. Partitions. Screens and dividers. Hunkering, clearing out, cramming, suspending. To push aside. To make room for and find that one can always live with less—clothing, time, breathing space. To find all along there has been room for another, to feel *increase* in the crowded space I am becoming.

Jed moved his work into the basement, and now one room is cleared and waiting. And emptied, it makes a clattering when my foot falls hard on the top stair or I enter quickly. For all the sound it collects, there is a stillness to the bare room; light through the window gathers precisely, and with less to fall on, pours, blossoms, and streams. It kicks itself wide. The bare room, slowly filling with light, with baby things, resembles the odd loneliness of a new friendship, softening. Through an accumulation of talk, by being together at different hours of the day, how the smallest moments accrete toward an intimacy. Yes, the room will be full again and the loud clattering subside, but for now, the spaciousness is remade with a thought: January: the room is a wide field in the country of the house; a snow, a hail is gathering, packing its gray force until the sky breaks open, over the expanse of this scuffed wooden floor we will pace and dance on, over sunspots and nightfall, to make a distance of our child's crying.

august 18

Late summer, so much catches the eye. All the heavy green fills the frame of the window, tangles in, and makes of the center pane a small clearing through which I can see weeds grown into the cracks in the steps, white stitches the white butterfly makes in air. Birch leaves flip over, go silver in the slanting sun. And always, when the long, loose vines dip beyond the tangled bush into clear space, I look up and out quickly, respond with immediacy to the movement that catches my eye, though I'm not able to say what I'm looking for or expecting. Instinctively my head pulls up to locate the disturbance, to attend, and yet there's nothing there beyond the circumscribed green, the prop of the moment and its clever gesture, designed, it seems, to snag, of all the indifference surrounding it, *my* eye, *my* care.

Perhaps distraction at its most fruitful is a state of richest expectation; or distraction visits when we are most accepting of imposition: are willingly drawn far from routine, invited out of step and consistency and into a puzzle, a puzzlement. Is there a first step one takes then, in belief, in the hope that interruption has with it a gift, is not merely the undermining of intention? Here comes the world suggesting itself, in this form, in that form, and at each turn a chance to adopt it anew, to follow its roots down and routes in.

Isn't this the action beginning, the conflict introduced to the placid-seeming moment? The grain of sand agitating toward its luminous, changed state? And isn't the only thing, then, to accept the mystery coming for you, breaking into your peace, into *mine*, because I am no longer audience but, moment to moment, protagonist, splintering away from the opening scenes, further into the act—and really what else could I do in this drama, watched as I am, by everything out there dipping, crawling, waving, pouring itself out in front of me? Opening, as I will open, into the singular moment.

august 21

Later today I will stand up to my ankles in a bed of ivy on the slope in the backyard, and tear climbing vines from the trunks of three close-set pines. The ground there is an overgrown snarl, so the ivy sought breathing space in air. Something lively in the patch of woods is shaking down pods or hitting one thing against another. A line of thunderstorms is moving through, the air weighted past lush, past pulsing, into these last weeks where growth is no longer a burgeoning but a teetering excess—a kind of spill, a lapse into spoilage and clabbered in the scent of itself. Even the green of new clover sinks into a darker bed of long grass, a tangle around it, which pulls like a tide. On a clear day at the end of November, light will brighten from further off, will come through high clouds as if pinched, as if trying. Already I am eager for the efforts of that light, for a brown tranquility, curled leaves, a conformity of whites and grays. But first the blaze.

august 29

We're waiting for a hurricane. Trees in a state of watchfulness exhale, and the humming current of cicadas rises when the wind thins. It's a nervous call-and-response out there, the limbs in parts thick and lush, in parts thinning and laced with brown, and I am, *we are* at the edge of it all, held back and listening into, not hearing the significant word or telling pause, but understanding more primitively the cadence of conversation, all tone and intent. Warnings: the car horn blaring and dying as it passes with urgency as if in a fog, out over water, jagged rock, and the darkening sky.

This early in fall, the air is all threshold, stubbornly unformed and resistant to shape. A splicing together—the warmth of indoors still on the body as, once outside, the cooler air presses slowly in. Sometimes pockets of air, patches of weather materialize, and it is as strange as coming upon a Japanese paper screen in the middle of a field, some small demarcation in a vaster space.

"You might be feeling anxiety, fear of the future, boredom with the subject of pregnancy in the sixth month," my guidebook says. Perhaps so, but I want to know *why*, and what are the origins of those generalized "feelings"? The simple affirmation of their free-floating quality isn't satisfying.

"You might continue to experience forgetfulness." I certainly have and it was frightening at first; I was succumbing, yes, but far more diminishing was the book's easy checklist of reassurances: "a lot on one's mind" and "a busy time." What is this breathing silence in the face of questions I haven't the scope to shape yet?

Arriving in a new place, you start from an acknowledgement of strangeness, a disciplined use of discomfort and surprise. Later, as observations accumulate, the awareness of contrast dwindles and must be replaced with a growing understanding of how observations fit together within a system unique to the other culture. Having made as much use as possible of the sense that everything is totally alien, you begin to experience, through increasing familiarity, the way in which everything makes sense within a new logic. Eventually an ethnographer will hope to develop a description of a whole way of life that will convey this internal consistency, in which the height and placement of a chair, the adult response to a crying baby and to voices raised in dispute and the rules about when to relax and the rhythms of the day can be integrated, although never perfectly.—Mary Catherine Bateson

It is exactly the friction of a new encounter, the dislocation of being in a new land, the noting and privileging of misalignment, and even the intrigue of discomfort, that makes learning possible. I'm finding that *advice* (a form of nostalgia in itself) to *take it easy* or *enjoy this time because you won't have it again* or the practical tips so many books offer discourage rigorous engagement. They certainly don't urge exploration of confusion, awe, or the wild swing between the two. Is this enormity, the psyche's and the body's, best described as a force to "relax into" rather than one to wrangle with, to form and shape, however partially?

Not naming or thrashing out what it is that distracts allows the atmosphere of this hovering time to remain a hazy numbness or to leak out in back-door ways. "You may be experiencing vivid, frightening dreams," another guide states, and indeed, the angular house we rented by the ocean—it was as stark there as December but uncomfortably warm—was slowly being absorbed by green, intoxicatingly green water rising on all sides, soaking the foundation, loosening it, the salty colloidal stir pressing against the glass walls as if the house itself were a fish in a tank and the animated water a threat peering in.

Drowned, overwhelmed, pulled under: all metaphors holding the place of a serviceable language. And so, to begin, a brief list of the unspoken, a clumsy net thrown into the dim pool: What if I don't like my child? What if he is unpleasing to me, as once, indeed, happened mightily, as in "and Cain was unpleasing to the Lord." And how was that fate explained to the child? God's random preference leaves us stumped, but a mother's love, unconditionally given, should surpass that of God? "What if I don't like being a mother?" That is, what if I can't reconstruct a life in which a known identity might resume? "My insufficiencies will ruin my child." And so on.

No wonder my guide poses in chapter 6, "At Six Months," this question: *Can't anyone think of anything else besides pregnancy?* Of course it wears thin as a constant topic of conversation, as do all predictable subjects and questions, but I think there is more of a plea behind the complaint—*Can't anyone talk to me about what we're not talking about? And why can't you, who have gone before me, speak what you know?* I've had enough of substitutions: Have you painted the room? Do you know the sex? The real longing I hear in the book's cranky phrasing is for a frank reassessment of the terms of our own conversion and conversation.

About the geneticist J. B. S. Haldane, Bateson recounts: "He was asked what, on the basis of his knowledge of the creation, he could infer about the mind of the Creator." His answer was surely revealing: "An inordinate fondness for beetles." Amusing. And true to his life's close work—but who, I wondered, thought to ask a man who studied *beetles* about the nature of creation?

Bateson again: "The eye of compassion is as rare and valuable as the beings for which that compassion is felt. Its sensitivities depend on picking out one pattern from the mass and recognizing a kinship to it."

What if we turned that compassionate eye, that delving, adventurous, partial-yet-searching eye out on ourselves, on our own experience as it is happening, or in reflection, or in anticipation of? To ask a woman—near giving birth, about to enter that long hall, or having done so years ago—what she might infer about the mind of the Creator . . . or, for that matter, what it is she sees now in the face of the rose beetle, the perfect triangle of the mantis's delicate, voracious head?

I heard this evening on the radio about the frigate bird, a majestic thing that makes its home in the West Indies and Brazil, and about how flocks of them with their abundantly long and colorful tail feathers are swept up in the gales of hurricanes and carried hundreds and sometimes thousands of miles and dumped inland in other countries. Some are so tired and emaciated that they soon die, while others take a few days to reorient, literally get their bearings, and then begin the long flight back. I tried to imagine those birds landing in a cornfield somewhere, far from their orange groves, their blue-green water and sweet fine sands. I tried to imagine picking up, intuiting home, and going, tracing back to a place I was pried from, not knowing how I got to the new land or even being able to gauge the distance I was tossed. I tried to imagine those long days and what I would need—the stamina, the compass, the plotting, the recovery, and the will.

august 30

I remember the insects, and when my sister, younger by two years, was still unafraid of the transformations from purple to black on the backs of beetles, of the lacy webbing of a mantis's wings and its intelligent, pearl-sized eyes, considering.

I remember she held something, one hot morning, between her fingers, a cricket or the parchment shell of a cicada, and showed it to me, or didn't show me, was simply walking around with it, and I told her to put it down, drop it, or worse, recoiled. I remember how she looked at me, surprised she had so misinterpreted, misgauged what to do with insects and how to feel about them. And then she *did* drop it. Soon after that, she began flinching at the same insects she had once held up to her eye or squatted over. She no longer raised them, plainly and gently, with a child's absorbed, blank attention. And I remember the sadness I felt, having taught my sister to flinch.

And yesterday afternoon, a downy woodpecker landed and walked along the stone steps, listening, then sank its long beak into a crack and pulled up sticky load after load from all the dark wetness in there; it was at its task a long time, never looking up, not fearing for itself in that twitching, cautious, birdlike way. The light doused the steps and the bird was out in the open, itself spotted with light. It must have been overcome: everything it wanted, dark and sweet, rich and unguarded, there for the taking. Its languor made me forget it was a bird, with a bird's nerves, and hollow bones, a heart of fear calibrated for flight. I think its lids must've been lowered in rapture, because no distraction at all could counter the day, the sunny patch where it bobbed and rose, the dark abundance of the cracked stone, that deep well, would it ever stop giving?

september 9

Laid out perfectly where they fell in the tall grass, half sunk in
the soft ground—the bones of a small cat. And how long did it
take for the bones to clean, for the flesh to slip off and the eyes
burn away? The shape the body made was placid-seeming,
unlike the animals of prehistory, who, trapped in tar in the
posture of shock, in half-light on a cave wall, are forever
outrunning fire, weather, attack. In caves their broad, simple
bodies are sketched in ochre flight; fear is the black cipher of
an open mouth, the red oxide smudge on a flank. But I found
these bones in the shape of sleep, of full and open expectancy,
mid-stride in an airy leap. *Waiting for.* I learned it takes only
days for a small animal's body to decompose at this time of
year, to return itself to bone, to its simplest components—
carbon, hydrogen, oxygen, nitrogen, sulfur. To press its outline
back into the soft earth, which is a welcoming, rich place still,
late summer. A home receiving the body in, expecting it.

september 10

Four workmen, one very short, walk together up the long hill.
Three outstrip the smaller one, who takes the incline double-
time. And I do not think *why aren't they slowing* but instead
am convinced that they couldn't have slowed. That would've
been pity—they'd be guilty of pity, and somehow then,
complicitous with the fate that granted their height and left
him small. They'd have to acknowledge fate's unfairness, and

their own inability to alter its plot. Not waiting for him maintained an intactness, theirs, and perhaps his: Let us agree to ignore the randomness that makes us all. Let us not surrender to the need for contingencies, or admit we have only smallest power to alleviate some of the suffering, some of the shock which, daily, dulls and drains the spirit. Let us not be meek at all. Let us not inherit anything that calls for return, concession by concession. Let us not admit we are dwarfed by the speed of horses; we do not count that difference as cause for shame. Let us ignore the relief we won't speak of, how even our kindness is weighted against that terrible moment of gratitude—*I am not he*. And let us admit, too, the fear of receiving another's mediating kindness.

Perhaps we are made whole for a reason; without such intent, we are likelihood and whim; each a gratuity. And so, may those of us who are whole know this: the caprice of our bodies goes mercifully uncataloged by a public eye. May we fear the hidden, dark flaws that cause no one, yet, to slow for us. Let it be known that the three men are otherwise good to the fourth, natural-seeming, and behave with equanimity.

Let me withstand the vulnerabilities of my child, and not because I can anticipate his rapid changes, growing strength, his growing safely away from us. But let my child, small as he is, as he might always be, stand before me in his need—I who could not help him to grow, were he not meant to, any more than I could help him to . . . and here I cannot come up with one thing more I couldn't do for my child, if I just tried hard enough.

The rain this afternoon and now this evening is cool and
slaking; it turns the seasons over. Throughout the afternoon
the rain strengthened and, opening the door of my office, out
into the wet, my feet cold in sandals, I walked home in it, past
the heavy, nearly frightening sunflowers next to the dumpster
at the edge of campus. How deeply they were bent by the
weight of their dripping faces. Then I was dry, and at home
cutting eggplant, stripping the purple skin in even lines,
when Jed came and looked out the back door and said,
"There's our rabbit." Possessive because we've watched her
grow; ours because she chose us, kept us in sight all summer,
and how many times was distracted by our kitchen light
flicked on or off? How often had she stopped munching a root
and lifted her head to watch our progressions through a
window?

She was sitting in a little bower of vines, protected from the
hard rain, breaking off greens at their base and chewing them,
pulling them into her mouth with neat puckers. Her neck was
thicker and her movements slower, more measured than
earlier this summer. We watched as she sat and began to wash
off—first her face, then her whole head, both creamy front
paws drawn up and over her big ears, slicking them, then
fluffing the damp fur.

Throughout my own preparations, peeling and pressing
garlic and dosing in cumin, salt, and lemon, she stayed,
watching and chewing. I thought she'd make bare the patch
under the bush where she pulled up greens. I thought I'd

throw a lettuce heart out to her but knew she had all she needed within reach, and that yanking the swollen door open would frighten her away. So we stood, then I stood, after Jed left for rehearsal, and watched her through the window, full and finishing. She grew still and then twitched, twisted fully around, caught a whiff of something, drew up on her haunches and was gone. But where would she be safer, more hidden? I turned back to cooking, back to something I'd just read, a rabbi's commentary on the limits of prayer: should you, while walking home one day, see in the distance a house on fire, you may not pray, *Let it not be my house burning.* This would represent two concomitant evils: an implied wish that it be another's house burning, and an affront to the reality you see before you: a house, clearly, is already burning. So what to hope, then, running breathlessly closer? What state of regard to train on the scene, what mindful faith or desire compose in your flight toward the flames?

For all its very real limitations—foxes, cars, illness, poison— the thought "I hope nothing happens to our rabbit" is calming. I, who am big, unable to move as quickly as before and yet am conducted easily on, led, pointed toward; I who am so plainly *here,* and am also of the spate *out there:* the droves, the scrying, the profligate clacking. I was soaked by the time I got home this afternoon: remember that in the body, the cold, the wet. Remember the flame under the pot is contained. That my house is nowhere burning and I do not know then what prayer to make, every safe thing inexorably in motion.

Jed dreamed of catching the mouse we've seen—with his bare hands and trying to show, in some way, that he wouldn't close his fist over it or hurt it. And later, we did find, behind the old black piano, a nest of newborn mice. We scooped it up whole, put it in a shoebox and reset the Hav-a-Heart traps for the mother, hoping to relocate them all, but she wouldn't return. Not for food, or darkness, or silence (we drew the shades when we left) or the sounds of her hungry young. The hours passed, for them, without proper warmth or food. The SPCA said they'd take all eight but would have to put them to sleep. A stupid waste, we thought, and couldn't justify housecleaning that way, so we took the number of a woman who ran, from her home, a wildlife refuge center. Jed called and listened to the complicated routine Gerta suggested for saving the mice, which included stroking the newborn's bellies with a Q-tip dipped in warm water to encourage them to urinate before feeding. Feeding meant administering Pedialyte (we'd never heard of it) though tiny eyedroppers (though she doubted we'd find ones small enough) every few hours. We were dismayed and sounded, I feared, simply too busy to take proper care. She would hear it in our hesitation, would guess at our future as parents.

Gerta offered to take the mice, so we drove them out to her immediately. It took nearly an hour through the center of the city, east to a small, worn neighborhood near the docks. The pups, who had looked fresh and pink just an hour ago, now seemed shivery, gray, insubstantial. When we arrived, she met us in a flowered housedress, ready with a warmed, cotton-filled bowl. Talking with her, we learned that the mother wouldn't ever have returned to a place of such danger. She said she'd put the babies right away in a tiny incubator she improvised, and she carried them into the house close to her body, past the recovering hawk on a perch, its wing bandaged after flying into barbed wire; past the litter of rabbits, one-legged pigeons, a squirrel resting after a concussion. Cats with frayed tails and three angry opossums. Saint Gertrude, patron of mouse and rat catchers, who banished hoards from infested towns, who appears in portraits with mice running up and down her mild-looking distaff—passing her foxes, chipmunks, and ducks. Passing the curled and sleeping barn snake, the tall cage of the snowy owl who makes of anything it finds and eats, an astonishingly clean knot of bones.

october 2

I lift my shirt and look down, just to see your arm or leg move, graze my stomach from within. Or to see you reach for your ceiling, your soft tent, and make a moving roof of me. Or to watch you shift the entire mountain of my belly from its base, seismically tilt the whole floor of this sea.

I walked today, my usual hour of brisk recovery after teaching, through campus to the tulip garden, now, in the fall, replenished with mums and zinnias and hardy, faded-looking asters. The heavy heads of sunflowers were picked clean and hung from dry, fibrous stalks. And as my body hurt, the ligaments stretching, pulling like stitches across the expanse of me, I kept walking. Someone had tied, around the trunks of the biggest oaks in the park, hand-lettered signs that read "Caution: Beehives." *So I won't climb today,* I thought. I stood below the fanned skirt of one of the trees and looked up into the limbs, into the thick clusters of acorns and still-green leaves, but saw nothing. And heard nothing. Already the bees were driving down to the hollow parts, getting ready to sleep long months. They were deep inside, but I could see where they'd enter and leave again, being the live pulse of blood they were, the yellow rivulets of speech and hum guided by instinct into sweetness, into a rage as long as a black silk scarf in wind. Each with its job and the means to sustain itself and a household. I thought of the whole stutter of them *in there.* The entire proclamation they were. I kept walking and aching, around and around the long block, over the old sidewalks buckled by roots. I stepped over the jutting wedges of concrete, and over the burnished acorns that could trip me up—it would take just one underfoot and I'd go down, onto the mossy path, slick leaves and patched sun. My hands were swollen and uncomfortably tight and hot in the brisk air. I was passing the grayed face of the dog behind its wrought iron fence, the gathering squirrels, the nanny or babysitter walking the bundled children in the middle of the day; I was passing the children's secret feelings about her, her perfume, accent, the hint of impatience that might sound simply musical to anyone else, and the stitch in my side was going, replaced by a muscle tensing and strengthening, finding a gait that would sustain me. I kept walking, more solidly, back into my body,

past you and the discomfort of carrying, back to myself,
around the block of huge houses again, and once more, back
into a body that carries itself—and you came along too. Kept
coming along.

october 3

The ghost I met when I lived in Poland was an old woman.
She wore a black dress that morning, in the cold, turn-of-the-
century apartment where we stayed, in Bydgoszcz, for a short
time. I passed her on my long walk to the bathroom when the
early dark was just spooling up. A ghost is a marvel, or a
marvelous moment: it makes disappear the occasions for
language, encourages a nimble hiatus across which understanding skips. For a reason, I'm sure, I was all apology as I
bent to the loud faucets to wash. I awaited her judgment. Sheer
as she was, I could have wished her away, my hand through the
air, scattering the light, the breath that composed her. But I
was still; not *held* still, but arrayed in the quiet she was. Then,
I knew she knew how I loved to inspect the apartment's old
organ, half draped in heavy, red velvet in the long hall; I knew
she saw me pause, just this morning, just briefly in the cold on
my way to the bathroom, to see again the pearled knobs, the
dusty keys and brass pedals, and the names of each voice
calligraphed in Italian, in gold on the stops. She spoke, too, in
the grace of a long curtain in wind, then turned entirely to
light and was gone. What she allowed was my presence, that
I might stay in her house. I who turned my face into the
running water in response.

october 22

The angel in the postcard tacked on the wall is leading the boy and girl across a steep wooden bridge—it must be one side paradise, one side earth. She's hovering over them as they manage, wobbly and cautious it seems from this angle, as I lie heavily on my back, feet propped, looking up from a book. Hers is the face of a woman bent to her task, a very real woman who is, nonetheless, like the water below the children or the sky above them, also a presence, an atmosphere informing their journey. Lips parted the way her green robe parts in air. She is a breath herself, such a pale blue she's almost white, sparest sky or rain-washed brightness. The children are crossing to safety. Care darkens her eyes, her robe unfurls, her long hair falls from the tilt of her head, and she whispers over the children, cold vapors of morning, the puff of breath visible now that it's fall, now that it's taking them so long to cross, fixed as they are in the middle of the picture.

When I put my hand down to feel your kicking, you stop, and when I take my hand away, you start again. How could you know my intention? My child, I make a decision: not to think you are either soothed by my touch and so stop kicking, or are already sly and independent, refusing anyone's terms but your own. I cannot know what you are or will be; instead, you will surprise me, and I, quick as your kick and your quieting, will reach down and surprise you—my hand on your arm, leg, or shoulder. *There.*

Outside, the tail of a storm is passing, trees and wind, wind and trees reaching and swatting. Each one's movement proves the other's existence. One bends deeply and the other sighs.

october 23

My hand on your arm or leg or shoulder: the only hand I will lay on you. One that, for you, will learn better the nature, the limits, the possibilities of anything at all—cloth, paper, flesh, fear; a hand that goes simply to the task: peeling an orange, untangling thread, knotting, plaiting, slicing, pouring, turning pages; a hand with the knowledge of a head's sleeping weight; one that won't in frustration force keys, twist badly threaded lids, or leave the toothpaste cap half-turned; a hand that maintains in its gestures a belief that the world speaks through its objects; fluent, with a life apart from the body's, a hand not merely annexed to the body, attached to the long crane of the arm and limited by its big steering motions; hand of the mind, with a mind of lilacs, scenting the air around it; of hair when absently twining hair; of stone when it turns the stone over to regard the cool, water-stained underside. A hand that will make of an empty soup can a hat, a bank, an animal's ribbed body, a wheel, a house, music.

november 1

I can see through the towering azaleas now, straight through the clumps of wisteria that hung all summer like the tongues of great bells, or softened bunches of grapes, humming with sweetness. There's Mary, familiar as any neighbor known at a distance, noted in passing. She stands ankle-deep in pachysandra in the yard. She's holding, I used to think, tucked back from the alley in her little grotto, fistfuls of her long stone skirt. That she had gathered up the material and was holding it, bunched, ever about to take a step. But she's balancing, now, handfuls of soft snow. Snow melts on the ground, settles on her palms, upturned. Above her, the arc of magnolia is all ribs and bare limbs, black in the damp as the fresh snow lofts down, and she's getting a little cap too.

I was here, in this spot, one day last spring, in weather so beautiful it bent her over. Wilted, she seemed, in her heavy garments, in sun. A thick stone hem pulling her down. Slope-shouldered, she strained forward to ease the cloak from her forehead. The clouds moved fast, and when I turned toward home, the rain came on. The rain pulsed down and the wide concrete alley cooked up a vapor that sizzled and rose and broke apart. The rain came faster and the sky tipped more steeply, a dark meniscus sliding to a pour.

Mary was soaked but not *caught* in rain. Hard to say why, when everything breathed its surprise at the quick change— people ducking indoors, birds lifting high into sheltering crooks. She was, instead, catching it. Lightning tore down and the noise of roiling currents moved over. Shards of, needles of rain were landing. The construction crew nearby smiled; smiled and slowed. One drop hit my scalp, came cleanly through my hair. It was cold and precise, then my head was wet, and rain was trickling onto my face. The force of the rain turned my green shirt black. I slowed further, and then, still blocks from home, I, too, turned my palms up. In a minute more, I would be soaked through completely. And without a thought, I turned my palms up. The rain had me do it. The workmen stood, as I did, in the torrent—with no cover, what else could they do? But Mary's palms, just so, in perpetual storm. It was perpetual rain she was catching—was not *caught in,* but stood under, hands up, receiving.

november 22

Don't leave, I want to say. *Stay in.* I want to keep you as close as thought, as undercurrent, *sotto voce,* the secret pronunciation I have for certain words: wrong, I know, but familiar as dialect, the way I first read and learned them. I have come to know you in your silence, hidden behind the heavy curtain I am. Days and nights we wait for you, this waiting a way I'm reluctant to give up. I am reluctant to give up the slant of this time, the sharp angle of sun going down on rich grain, that plank of sun just so through the pane, that the potted violet might rest on the warmed sill. I want always to be angled so, toward the world, in the late afternoon of the moment, the object of its most ardent gaze and perfect illumination. I want to still this time, which holds its own passing as close as a skirt hitched before the step up and over the threshold, this steep pause of months, gathered and piled. This time is an exhalation of light at rest on a chin, now a neck and lower, lower, now upon you, our child, where once it burnished only my cheekbone, gilded only my hair. And already it is underfoot, slackening, untwining, passing into a hardy dusk. Rounding. Gaining on. A day is coming with a name for all I cannot hold off saying much longer.

december 1

All the words that sketch a place, clearly and singularly in the mind, begin to merge the closer one draws to the destination. Facts untether and disembody in the face of the scene, the seen, the arrival. Reading about the place I am becoming has been something like consulting a travel guide. Words are signs for upcoming vistas, mile markers to follow: *Stare Miasto*, the Old City in Warsaw, *this way*. But then the slowed looking comes: the crumbling ramparts crumble daily; geese peck at crusts in the palace gardens. Smaller, concentric geographies abound: flower stand, apothecary, baking tins in Marie Curie's childhood home—all of which alter the monolith of "destination." Any journey might be prefigured by a guide. But even the most precise itinerary carries within it a secret heart of distraction: there will be, along the way, a crow tearing at the pale ribs of a deer. A wild clash of honeysuckle, vines buckling with scent, and that secret drop of nectar to pull up in the stamen's little bucket and touch to the tongue.

Headache, hunger, elation, *exhaustion:* words veer, directionless.

For a few weeks, early on, mine was an exhaustion so profound, so narcotic, that surveying my thickening body, it seemed to bypass that larger mass and go to work directly on the brain, sending from an isolated control station an all-points-bulletin of torpor. I couldn't move. Around that time, at three months, I read about the chemistry of exhaustion, about what was released when into the stream of fluids I shared with the child, and what was carried away. At first glance, *exhaustion* referred to a common seeping out and down—to be wrung, as after a day-long hike. But the sleep I fell into—a stop and give-over affair—had nothing to do with the slow drip of anything, nothing to do with the word *exhaustion* itself, which spoken aloud sounded lighter than air. What I felt weighed in like a boulder—no warm pour of molasses or haycock softening gold in sun. It was a rough-faced slab—not even granite, all faceted and internally jigging with light—but cold, elementally present, immobile, imposing. Not even stubborn, for that implies an active stance taken, a counterforce applied. This was a finality, an outer edge. Refusal absolute and clarity so stark it was nearly moral: truth so unmistakable I could sharpen my powers of intuition on it. It spoke and I had to listen.

Early on, *exhaustion* was a cipher on paper. It meant, "You'll be tired." At nine months now, I layer the word. I let it resound beyond its near borders, written lowercase, with its two spires, smokestacks, tallest trees above the undergrowth of vowels. The word now is a sign for a lived physicality, the truth of the body. Other words, too, have changed, flowered, imploded, solidified—no—slipped their skins, slipped off the page in the night to gather more wilderness into their veins. Veins—still perfect or badly constructed, *swelling, spidering, varicose.* Like *exhaustion,* those words do not become more precise, perceptive small selves on their own. Rather, we've established a familiarity together; there is a deepening between us. A word's tone, flex, and impulse, its mark, flavor, implications, shade, and taint, are altered by the self I bring along to its banks. Its

reedy, overgrown, seething banks. That boundary, where
ghosted things sing, multiply, breathe, then suddenly hold
their breath in fear, until the long shadow of the reader passes.

It passes.

They are richer, full of bravado, enlivened. Alive.

More words stream forth in their thin, worn garments:
contraction, dilation. More pilgrim selves at arm's length—
solitary, suggestive. More mile markers and these last slow
months a Kansas, a Texas: so much plain space. Until months
later, I will return to these words—complicated and roughed
up—to read in them their stories, the colors of nurses' smocks,
chipped ice in cups, chopped ice in neat mounds in the black
parking lot. Late winter's sharp angle of light into which
someone's cries will come.

december 31

I am given a polished brass key, a packet of salt, bread, a red
silk ribbon tied in a loose knot I am meant to unbind. I am
told to unbraid my hair and remove the silver clip I wear.
Unlock the doors and windows and an easy labor will be mine.

I put the beautiful old key in my pocket, use the salt at
dinner and the bit of crusty bread too. I untie the ribbon and
draw it between thumb and forefinger a few times for the
good, cool pull. I brush my loose hair and unlock—then
quietly lock again—the front door against the cold.

january 3

The baby should be here in a week. There are children abounding. Standing like cornstalks, poking like sun rays from a fiery center. Children like hours, so many set neatly around in a circle. Each pointed to with a thin, shapely hand. Seconds of children. The ticking increases: children like years, millions, but *this* one, this year, into which my child was born. Rain, but the drop that landed neatly in *my* eye. So that I am blinking, surfacing now, into dark January's cold light. I'm not sleeping these days which are nights. Which are days like no others. There is nothing more rousing or conclusive than this: *this is happening to me*, which means I am not, in any way, alone.

january 15

Our baby is late by a week—or not. How can we know its plan, the plan, really, that is not even its own? No one knows what triggers birth, or even what sets this amaryllis to growing *now* and *in this light*, at this temperature and not another, not resting another year, or flowering in earnest in false spring: here, in its deep, red heart, the trumpet sound is being born. There is the mind of something other inside me—not the child's, for that mind is hardly made up, its very bones unsealed, unplaited for months to come, still thickening like the crust on a bread. The birth will be made to happen in a week if it doesn't begin on its own.

To acknowledge the mind of the body, the biological mind and its decisions, is as slippery as acknowledging the mind of aesthetics and its choices.

I mean this: I imagine, the slow drip of oxytocin into the veins, initiated, it is now believed, by hormones released by the hungry baby who needs more nutrients than the mother can supply. Yet how does hunger make itself known—not at one discrete moment, but then suddenly, at the next. It comes on. Like a gas it seeps. Like a dampness it flowers and laves and plumes—and suddenly, you *are*. Ravenous. Of a single mind.

There is a beautiful, impossible Zen koan—"Show me your original face, the face you had before your parents were born." It is close to the question physicists work toward: What was there before there was something? What popped, or poured, sprung, dazzled, so necessarily, so extravagantly, that one hydrogen atom into being? Or better still, why? A hunger, a pang, a craving for? An aesthetic is not a taxonomy.

We have—and this notion is so mysteriously simple— a bent, a leaning, an inclination toward—a redder red, one not so orangey, not quite rusty, more a barn's, no—love's flush, no—anger's boil; *this* red. That's it! *It strikes us,* we say, as authentic, provocative, lyrical. Newly or familiarly. With glacial poise. With human warmth. Cooked or raw. Just because. And so it goes around the dinner table, around and around. At Wallace Stevens's it goes like this:

Table Talk

Granted, we die for good.
Life, then, is largely a thing
Of happens to like, not should.

And that, too, granted, why
Do I happen to like red bush,
Gray grass and green-gray sky?

What else remains? But red,
Gray, green, why those of all?
That is not what I said:

Not those of all. But those.
One likes what one happens to like.
One likes the way red grows.

It cannot matter at all.
Happens to like is one
Of the ways things happen to fall.

    I do not want the birth induced. I understand, of course, why it is done—to prevent contact with a deteriorating environment. I understand. I've marked the calendar with that final date. But I want the thought of the mind of my body to retain its own shape, its elegance; indeed physicists reject workable theories, dislike them solely because they are not subtle, not ample, too encumbered. Not *it.*
    I want the thought to complete itself, not go on and on as a drone—that unstoppered rush of air in bagpipes, in a pipe organ before the tune is made, is sculpted by the muscular

press up and down the dark tunnel. I want the body to know, to feel for the right time, have its timing, a sense of tempo. A sense of phase and phrase and a way to express it.

I'm thinking of the old cartoon in which some character, at the end, zips up the whole screen, the landscape, the story, himself included, and the show is over. How tidy and complete it was. How improbable the gesture. And how I *liked* that.

birth) *january* 16, 1997

january 20

Days and nights of sensation so furious I must, before entering
this time fully, cast back. Or rather, it is more *up* I should go,
into a clearer element, before I drop wholly back into the
dense, strange now. I balance for just a little longer, Joseph and
this past, what I want to remember of it:

The queasiness: not out-and-out sickness but a slant vertigo
of the whole body, which tried to locate a middle, a crowded
safe ground, where it might settle and churn a simple gyre.
Predictably, it arrived in the third month; unpredictably, it was
not a stone rushing through currents, but a wandering out
from under, something loosed seeking attachment in my body.
And though the sensation registered deep within, its force was
irresolute at first, and so I tried to keep it down, press or quiet
it back. There was hunger but little desire to eat, to tether
myself to the earth. I wanted instead to join the sway, to swim
with the fast riptide and be carried out far. And then, tired of
the back and forth of it all, dizzy, not dizzy, I wanted just to
stand upright, in shallow, knee-high eddies. I was growing
heavier, but my center was seafoam, home to a thing smaller
and lighter than a clot of wet sand.

The pains: I'd think of them cartographically, like the quick
dips and rises of a green contour map. One came as a pressure,
another as jostlings, like being pummeled from within;

I remember thinking *Is that my spleen the child's found?*
I remember his foot wedged under my rib: impossible to
bend forward, as if holding a dictionary to my chest while
trying to reach down for something I dropped. Another felt
as if my bladder was being squeezed like a lemon, which made
me laugh—what did, the sensation or the image? There was
the way the pelvic muscles, once finally relaxed in sleep, had to
contract to pull me upright many times a night. The sensation
of attenuation, the ropy ligaments, smooth as taut skeins of
silk, winching a great weight closer and closer to an edge.

The aches from his kicking and my own insomniac
writhing, from our turning and flipping, his funny hiccups.
The whole range of me shifting like a tilt-a-whirl floor. Joseph
moving like a hand under a tent, a shadow puppet, small head
under a blanket, that makeshift house.

One night—only one—of crushing, searing heartburn.
Of corrosive eddies around the breast bone for hours. And a
night of leg cramps, as if I'd swum miles in the salty dark and
the water suddenly froze around me.

I write back to the discomfort to alloy, in my body, the
events just before Joseph's arrival. I do not want to believe that
the fabled loss of the memory of these pains, and birth's pain,
has an evolutionary advantage at all, that forgetting, as one
doctor wrote, ensures the continuation of the species.
Something more lasting must ensure that, something from a
woman's mouth, straying out beyond, but inclusive of the
primitive "*Oh*" of pain. It seems likely that the difficulty a
woman experiences in recounting birth has much in common

with the difficulties she has, daily, of writing after that birth. If one cannot practice seizing moments, is not encouraged to receive and then note, is not given the time; if the event of sitting down to is not habitual and others are not habituated to it, then any experience soon loses its footing, dissolves into musing. The atmosphere of the event remains, with its broad designs—the recollection that "it hurt"—and perhaps an odd scrap of detail—"there was that bright light in my eyes"—but the wholly singular route into the event is gone: how in the labor room there was no mirror and you didn't miss it, how the clock was positioned immediately in front of you and you wanted it gone, time rearing up as it did, on its own; how shiny the sharp-edged steel cabinets, and who climbed up to clean them? The taste of the awful, pure oxygen you were made to breathe and the heat of the mask strapped to your face, for just a minute, until you shook it off . . .

There was the daily dropping and rising, his dropping in free-falls, your push up from a soft chair. There was the thought of yourself as doubled, calling you back from solitude. The lolling and swimming in the dark pond at night, yourself a dark pond. Meeting resistance and pushing against it, pushing against the steering wheel to get out of the car, pushing hard against the heavy front door, pushing and pushing, until you pushed yourself back, into your own tired body.

january 30

Here is the X of his crossed feet in sleep: crossed as the rich do, poolside in their chaise, as the poor do on their stoops in the heavy heat. Crossed, as all of us do, in sleep, fireside, or at the dock's edge. Intuitive crossing of currents there, the left learning the ways of the right; at the soft hillock of the ankle bone, the electrical snap, where, skin on skin, the charge jumps tracks; prongs of the divining rod overlapped near springs; the tips of calipers resting. Black inky footprints, a new sign to go by; prints with lines, mounts and valleys, planes, stars, pits, and islands—all clearly stamped on the creamy white card Jed carried at the hospital to identify himself as Father.

And fingers, too; the left hand with its ring finger, believed to cure wounds by mere touch. The index finger, perfect and wrinkled, which must not be pointed at a flowering orchard lest the fruit therein wither and die. A waving finger, which, right now, cannot find the mouth that wants to suck it, much less an orchard, or the perfect skin of a single peach.

february 3

When he sleeps for hours, this visitation comes: the desire for his crying and for the chance to comfort, to feel the distress in his breathing becalmed. Restorative to feel for another, for their body, which is only one's own body gone beyond itself again: black body of the crow as it walks on the asphalt: how good the rough scratch and tug on sharp claws. And the sharp jerk of the gray squirrel's head: how quickly it refocuses its eye, the size of a cowpea, a pigeon pea, but seal black, black as a blood clot. And the fern's tight coil late at night, early morning: a doubling over, hard laughter, a fist. A dry leaf skittering across the street: fear as I've known it, rushing through like ill wind. And of the mourning dove's shell pink and gray, velvet brown, lichen green breast: for an approximate, go just past the liver, go lightly in and there is the gall bladder similarly hued, below a pale scrim of ligaments. Go to the whole body hanging over the child for the churn, the workings of the mourning dove's song, for its sweet and desolate five-note song.

)))

These first weeks with him at home recall my first days in other countries where I've lived—that initial fear of venturing out alone, without a full and fluent language to navigate the way; and though the reticence of these past weeks has much to do with discomfort, with not being physically able to move around quickly, there is the same sense of holing up against fear, the fear calmed and reasoned with in overheated rooms, the craving for tea and sour bread with honey. And then, too, just yesterday, as I did one fall afternoon soon after arriving in Warsaw, I went out on my own. With Joseph now, in the sling, watching the shadows and leaves, whole trees going past, above in an arch, and me watching it all too, looking down and then up, seeing what he saw, trying to stay upright and not stumble in my distraction, cautious of the ache in my weak ankle as I took full, long strides.

Around the first corner, a supervisor rating our mail carrier. The dry, scrubby beaten yards, torn by children and dogs. An old, very old, shy woman walking with an aide and silver-wheeled walker—taking advantage of the warm, clear weather, the event the weather must have been for her, an event in which this new mother said hello and showed her baby and said how glad she, too, was for the bright day.

)))

At one month already his voice clarifies, his hands open from their tight curl and flatten in air. How to look, he shows us, with such open eyes and how to be held by a blackness and a whiteness, in the frill of green until it releases you, and you break off crying for want of more, from being too much, too terrifically filled.

)))

Though I go out regularly now with Joseph, I still cannot focus on objects at a distance. Even the images that come to circle him are drawn from a too-familiar storehouse: gold-edged and -leafed, filled with winged movement, touched with the miraculous light someone—Titian, Caravaggio, Vermeer— taught us to see. All I see and focus on is fine and precise; it occurs within a six-inch spill in front of me. Clear object after object comes, but close up, and only in the shapes he offers: the curve of his eyelashes. And not having *seen* much else recently, I have to think to find parallels: *as gently fringed as the antennae of the luna moth, as a watercolor brush feathering the green arcs of a fern.* And the color—*dried peat, maple syrup, chestnut.*

Beyond, the distance is a featureless space, and occurrences there, movement and color at its perimeter, are shapes without names. And closing that distance, I walk right past them, miracle that I am one body again, that there is so little to me that I can draw a deep breath and expel it fully. And when I lift him up, away from me, he is crowned not by my heart or the two sloped petals of my lungs, but by the dark buds starting already, out here, these last days of cold before spring.

)))

I want to remember the efforts of labor: the effort of directing the force building in my face and chest down to my pelvis, and lower, and how I could do that only visually at first, by imagining the force as a column of mercury dropping. How, soon, I couldn't distinguish between the imagined body and the actual. I had to let the power slide down, to slip from the mind toward the unseen body; I had to slip thought through the loop of the body until the distinction frayed and all was a clench unraveling.

I had to work with more concentration than I'd ever gathered before, in a vastness that then washed all image away and left me with only sensation. Jed's close face counted my breaths, and then, finally laughing and losing count, broke from numbers into words. How like an apprentice I felt, as if I knew just enough to glimpse what was required of mortal strength and honed musculature, but couldn't respond with any kind of finesse to the demands of the craft. I thought I might do well if only I could practice. I wanted to practice, to try again that transferring, that harnessing. I felt I was

learning, but already I was in the middle of the event. Not a
moment for reflection, consideration, study. Just the work to
be done and, clumsily, *now*.

And then it was over. Perfectly over.

How fresh Joseph looked, without his name for just seconds,
like a shell washed up, slick, rounded and wet, just pulled from
the depths and dropped at the edge of the shore I was, while
the tide rode away, back into itself. How beautiful even then,
his thick curves, his black hair, his permanence here on the
other side of the known world.

february 15

How he pulls away from the breast and latches on again;
off and on; on for a long while; off. Then that funny grimace
when he's had enough, as if the milk had suddenly richened,
deepened and turned.

february 22

The game he plays with black-and-white cards Jed folded into
a crown: he hits the crown away with his little fist and we move
it back so he can do it again. He tries again and again, and in
this way the shape of a smile begins to form.

)))

This is the tearful cry that makes us, sometimes, laugh: *Lah,*

lah. Lah, lah. Evenings, he makes a refrain of it, on and on, a song without verses.

march 1

What our friend Josefina did for us during the week she visited: cooked, cleaned, washed dishes; washed clothes; ironed; demonstrated proper burping technique; urged patience; showed me how to pump milk and store it; made dessert; swept; took me to the store with Joseph. Chose the food while I watched him sleep, milk-saturated under the awful bright lights and frightening aisles of too much, too much of what is called abundance.

march 22

I want to remember that, long ago, I started with scoffing; that I was sorry for mothers whose babies made them feel important, who derived a sense of worth from mothering. I want to remember that babies weren't a rightful measure of one's importance in the world—not like one's work; not like others' appreciation of it. What has fallen away? How have these days become not a measure of, but worthy in, themselves?

"I am here," Czeslaw Milosz writes. "Those three words contain all that can be said—you begin with those words and you return to them. 'Here' means on this earth, on this continent and no other, in this city and no other, and in this epoch I call mine, this century, this year. I touch myself against the feeling that my own body is transient. This is all very fundamental, but, after all, the science of life depends on the gradual discovery of fundamental truths."

And how, how did it come to be that *I* was given to *him?*
)))
His slicked lips, pursed and dripping after feeding: it is the look of enough, without thought to the next time, whether it will come when needed, whether it will be there at all.
)))
How broadly he smiles, so delighted with himself, with the face in front of him in the mirror. He raises his shoulders, tucks his chin in and makes himself look bashful.

march 16

Joseph is two months old now, and I'm able to sit down to work for a bit longer. He is more measurable, dependable in his job of building a discernible day and night for himself.
)))
He sleeps with his arms bent and over his head, such a completely open, restful pose; or sometimes, with his arms thrown high in triumph, as if in a perpetual cheer. "Goodnight Moon," the book begins. Good night to the wet, hanging mittens, the comb and brush duo, flat on the page on the rickety night table. One of everything to be said goodnight to,

oh perfect attenuation the book knows: let the farewells go on
and on. Late at night, reading and calming, the moon is the
clock in the labor room. The room is all whiteness and steel
under lights. No light to see him coming by as I squeezed my
eyes shut and it was as dark as his dark passage. It was nearly
midnight then and no mittens, no cats, no sleep for hours. As
there will be no sleep for hours here, and now, it looks like.

april 17

Our rabbit returned, or this rabbit is a ghost of the first, child
of the third, of how many rabbits is it now, in this one body,
stoutly up on its haunches out in the open, tallest rabbit ever,
ours grown this big, this quickly, it can't be.
)))
Sunlight passes through the aloe's thick leaves, and they are lit;
I am feeding my child, watching this, resembling it and not
knowing how. I reach down and touch what I think is satin, the
cool satin sewn to the edge of the wool blanket, but it moves
and turns as he turns, and I see it is his cheek.
)))
The light is laid out in squares on the floor and the child
who is already himself rests in my lap, feeding. We are sewn
together with needles of milk, with questions embellished—*is
he getting enough, how is it possible with such tiny sips*—and
assurances cross-stitched—*of course he is, look at him growing,
look at his legs hanging, already, over the edge of my lap.*
How unexpected to feel proud of his growing.

Thus the hours verge and converge on a certainty, which is also certainty of another kind: already he's out of his softest white sleeper; his mouth is no longer the silk knot of an infant's, but one that opens with intention into a laugh. And today when he woke after a long morning nap, I was startled, nearly frightened to see him distinctly older than he was just an hour ago. As if, because of a careless, greedy wish, because of a willful girl's desire, the new child were changed, as it happens in fables, into a beautiful animal which turns and runs hastily away.

m a y 3

The dove stretched for nothing, for joy, and revealed the white damask of its underwing and then drew its brown wings together again and folded into sleep. Mouse brown, fawn brown, and nothing like either animal, though as soft as they are if not fast. If not skipping or darting, though there's always a way to align oneself with, to soak each sheer face with the likeness of another.

If one can switch the time of day, exchange the burnishing light of morning, which makes a simple dish of a pond, with the light of dusk which releases the ruck of industry at the pond's edge . . . if one can see in the vine's tendril, in a vein of ore, a taut and held tension . . . bird's wings as bare shoulders, small ghosted forms that suggest a man reaching . . . how the quick dip in a child's clavicle suggests the bird pecking or recalls the bearing of a hawk catching updrafts and entering the woods with a pure and a cruel hunger . . . if one can see the desire to dig rocks and fill a pail with them, mix with a stick and the stick as a spoon, the sand as spice, the wind blowing, the mouth blowing to cool the soup off, then sit with that hunger at the long table you've filled and eat.

m a y 4

In college, where it was possible to study feminism, I learned this: I was never to *say*, though my body might one day bear life and be tethered to it for some time (for how long the tethering would go on was not studied), I was never to feel, though I might one day be lost in another's needs, might even have chosen to invite those needs—that by becoming pregnant I was partaking in a primal event. I was not to link myself to the myth of primitivism, to the earthbound quality of "women's knowledge."

What was this primitivism, really?—a way of being that was so elementary that we'd grown beyond it, evolved far past it? Though surely I hadn't experienced anything conclusively primitive about my body yet, nothing I could assuredly articulate and toss aside. This notion of my body as the site of a primal event could be used against me, I was told. As could any intrinsic quality ascribed to women: intuitive powers, earth-motherhood, the iconographies of *virgin, whore, martyr, siren*—see how much has already been mishandled by the patriarchy? Thus I was to be on guard against playing or being cast in any mythical role that tainted and corralled, controlled and objectified me, bequeathed me to a lesser realm, to a backward, nonrational self. My business was this: to fight my way into the light—Persephone scratching out her own maps on dark walls, plotting multiple routes, alternate endings. I was to be fierce and free, unfettered by my body, its mistakes, bad timing, or contingencies. Its wiles and drives were ownable. I was taught traps to avoid. I was taught a new destiny to wrangle with.

And for much of this clarity, for much of this context and articulation, I am thankful.

But some days, still, I am wholly unprepared for the joy of his scent, the slight arch of his foot at rest in my hand. I am unprepared for the power of delay: getting up from work to answer his hunger, returning to work with ideas springing, the edge of thought sharpened. So new is this *gathering* and *keeping*—and these the very words of a woman piecing scraps, putting up, putting by—that I am unprepared to be her: one woman with one man with one child.

m a y 5

I walked Joseph to the drugstore to get diapers: he wouldn't sleep and hardly ate, so, last measure, I took him out. No matter we'd been out all morning. He opened his eyes wide, staring up at trees, calming himself, and finally, on the way back, he slept. I think how, in recalling these small, spontaneous decisions years from now, I might, if not careful, represent them as intentional. *When he wouldn't sleep, I'd take him for a walk and he'd conk out* sounds so fixed, so full of certainty, tried and true, when in fact I have little idea of what will work, try the few tricks I know, try anything, just wing it.

He settles into routine then slips out of pattern so soon that I wonder if a routine really existed at all.

I would take him for a walk and he'd calm down . . . conveys nothing of his awesome, wordless preferences, how I felt about my dark hair shedding on all my clean white shirts, the shapeless headband I'd been wearing for months, for ease.

. . . and on the way back, he'd fall asleep: nothing of the frustration of arriving home and realizing I'd bought the scented baby wipes not the unscented, didn't get enough diapers, forgot that we've needed toothpaste for days now; nothing of the fact that the ugly jacket I'm wearing is too warm for this weather, is all I have with big, useful pockets; of how I'm still putting off going to the dentist and how each word and phrase collapses when I get them home and read the jottings I made on my notepad, how the air around the promising words stills, the pressure drops out from under and they lose all recognizable shape.

m a y 1 0

I am looking at *him. His* eyes with the green darts stirred into the brown. His fingers grazing air, then mine closing over them with a squeeze. The shape of his mouth forming conversation, one sound at a time; patches of hair curling and lifting in the breeze. The lines of his profile no sketch roughed in, but the slopes and curves light laves: all *Joseph*. There is nothing but specificity to gaze on, nothing of the leveling forces he will encounter. And what of the flinch I keep in check when doting men bounce him just a little too hard, say "Let's get out of here,

go for a walk, away from all these women." Do I release him
into the world of men, the place that assumes him and ferries
him out? Do I come along, follow at a distance, make of myself
the trail back? And as surely as Demeter must have each spring,
I feel the bloodline of fear enter and throb. Here, in this
stranger's land, how will I bargain for release of his body,
approach the forces that would steal him away, that would have
him labor under the will and eros of a masculine eye? What
wiles will I discover, and whose intercession will I seek to
broker a deal and return my boy?

This is not about keeping him young—small, dependable
and dependent, ensconced. It's about keeping him *away,* from
the elements of manhood that most resemble the dark of a
cave. But what more could Demeter have done? Stopped her
girl from gathering flowers that day, suppressed her growing
beauty, her curiosity, her play? Kept the corona of her hair
from unplaiting behind her in the breeze as she bent to study
the face of a flower or the jeweled back of a beetle in sun? Fixed
the way she possessed her own sex? And, as when nearing the
shore, the sharp-edged colors of sky and sea replace the
unshaped pour of atmosphere, so the roughness coming fast
to his body—on the skin of his hands from stroking and
clenching, on his cheeks chapping in wind—will, in some way,
without anyone's effort, make him recognizable as a man.

And should he be spirited away, for an hour, an afternoon,
to inhabit that world apart from women, what will he be asked
to give up? The preparation of food, as we are doing here, my
mother- and sisters-in-law and I? The choreography of talk
and readying, this ease of slicing and tasting, the mindless,

satisfying arrangement of reds and greens, and silver at the edges of plates? Though being jostled by men doesn't make him cry, neither does he seem to enjoy it as much as the songs his father plays and sings with him, or a bright puppet held out and made to dance wildly.

What will he do in that world of men? I cannot say I know. I cannot say I know the ways in which time spent there might be harmless, or engaging even. Or how, once there, jumping over fire, jumping over water, as so many boys have done before, the rituals of separation begin. I have only the knowledge of what he is urged to give up in order to enter that place. Of how he has already been asked to deny one for the other, the punishment for staying being branded a member of the clan of the feminine, which, defined as narrowly as it is by even well-intentioned men who want only to be close to my son, seems a wholly unattractive prospect to me, too. This invitation to join with men—in play, on a walk, wherever the "feminine" is absent, means, I fear, that my boy will turn from me before deciding how he himself might negotiate such divisions or live best in two worlds, entering, reentering, closing no door behind him.

And what am I then, should I openly mourn these divisions—overprotective? And thus implicated in his failure—and it is still seen like this—to grow up, to separate. Which is what it means, for many, to be a man. As if pulling him *in* or *back,* those spatial declarations of a woman's place, is a destructive act and not a rescue, not a return to the green world of light and burgeoning.

)))

Paging through a children's catalog: the girls' clothes are bright, theatrical, imitative of flowers and animals, with petaled collars and appliqued wings and ears, the spilled colors of high noon, the colors of burst pods and fully lush fields. Even the abstract ovals, the moon shapes, the platelets are bent head-to-head with their secrets. The boys' are duller, mown shades against such streak and dance, grounded skies darkened and loose weaves overcast, one shape in repose or a single bright shot. Theirs are clothes without frill or network, no eyeful, no blizzard of color. My little boy is meant already to restrain his palette, to leave the dazzle and shine to girls, to settle into narrower hues of expression, tempered and muted.

And how fleetingly, too, will his loveliness be enjoyed; how, even now, others qualify their enjoyment. Three or four times since his birth I've heard this: "He's so beautiful he could be a girl." And "Look at those eyes—wasted on a boy." The first time, as we were leaving the hospital and he was only days old. I still recall the look on the woman's face as she spoke, as we left the warm foyer and walked into the slate blue of that January afternoon with our new child—"Beautiful." And then, "Oh, it's a *boy*"—afraid she had offended me, yet unable to keep from commenting, from touching a finger to his dark, soft hair.

m a y 2 2

The raccoon is back: she's huge. I watched her climb a tree the other day in the middle of the afternoon, then hurry down and try the lids of garbage cans. And here I want so much to stretch into description—give the bulk of the animal wedged into the tree's dark crook, the color of its mask, not so black in daylight, more a deepening gray, almost a wetness splashed over the face, but I'm waiting for Joseph to wake up. The fussing I hear means any minute, or it means an hour from now he'll rise and I feel the space around my musing contract, cinch tighter with each moment like a puddle drying, and I'm daunted by the futility of entering the rich emptiness, the place of slow faith, where idea comes late, disguised as afterthought or near dismissal, where the raccoon crosses the street and ... then what? Finds and eats? Hides herself again? What would she do next?

I will need to be more cunning.

)))

We wonder again about her, she is out so often during the day. The neighborhood kids run screaming from the animal, adding to its strangeness. A neighbor says "I hope no one hurts it." Her husband says "She's just hungry." But it's the middle of the day. And how can she be hungry, I think, it's spring. She's fat with rats and garbage—and babies. That's easy to see. I'm annoyed at his diagnostic certainty, as if it's impossible to think she might be possessed by some wild, incalculable fever that drives her beyond her disposition, beyond her carefully cultivated, age-old raccoon traits, as she carries her young. As she carries her young, this fever is there, the terrible, complicated drive in her blood. It was there, too, in Sylvia Plath's drives to bear children, to write, to create in both arenas and simultaneously, to extinguish herself—nothing neatly arranged or divided, no easy diagnosis for hunger or fever, and all of it, all the dizzying exhaustion, the visitations of gift-words, whole poems, the urging toward sleep, peace, nothingness, all closing in at once.

I look at the heavy animal, its utter separateness as it climbs a tree nearer to the busy road than it's been before, everything delicately balanced on four small feet, back hunched as if against an anticipated blow. I do not think about calling the SPCA or animal control or any of the other helpful places suggested up and down the block. I think *she will flourish, and she will die*, that she knows this, proceeds with this knowledge, menacingly before us.

m a y 25

Joseph falls asleep listening to his parents laughing with their friends downstairs. I know this sensation, the smallness of my body, padded with familiar voices and the astonishing separateness that created. There is the world going on, going on without me. What it must be, for him, to be left for just a moment while I'm finishing up washing the dishes or forming a sentence. To be of your body and of the clean white of the wall—a white that, close up, unfocuses the eye so you swerve and falter in its wash. So you spin and cannot find proximity. How surprised he is when he looks up to see me again. How I don't exist at all for him, or, at times, for myself, when I'm gone from his sight.

)))

We never called to check on the baby mice we delivered to

Gerta in the fall, after all our effort, all our good intentions. We bought instead ten Hav-a-Heart traps in an attempt to catch the newest, wiliest one yet, with long ears, who leaves its droppings precisely around each trap but won't touch the cheese or peanut butter pushed inside. It's been months and we haven't yet caught it.

Late last night, after Jed washed the dishes away, I set up a barrage of traps on the stove and came down this morning to a wild clicking in one of them. Ate breakfast. Packed up the trap, packed Joseph in the car and drove to the reservoir to let the mouse go. As I lifted the trap door, it left slowly, cautiously, stepping onto the wet grass, darting a short distance, turning to see what brought it to this green place. Then, darkened with dew, it ran off. *Safe for now*, I thought, and *See it's gone*, I said to Joseph. But it was my own reprieve I was noting.

m a y 26

And let me remember, yes, *wanting* to be up with him, the exhaustion, the rocking, the unlikely solutions. I want to remember listening so closely to his cries that my throat would catch with his effort, and I'd gulp for more air, that holding him, my chest would vibrate as he drew in more breath. That the crying, so loud and so close, made a palpable shiver, like a seed rooting deep in my ear.

This is the method of countering pain that has always worked for me—to meet it without thought, to enter the seizing, the knotting, to breathe from within it. To be dimensionally drawn and contoured by it, a sculpted, single vertebra, peaked, gouged and planed, and organized around a central stem. How *he* would say it, the blue Buddha on the cover of my parents' book I looked at as a child: *Be Here Now*. I loved the separation of those three words, balanced around the rim of a circle, how spare and important they seemed, alone and together; how alone and together they formed both command and suggestion. I lean close and breathe in Joseph's seamless cries, swallow them, inhale, drape them over my shoulders, make a hood, a belt to pull tighter, an elixir which turns me drowsy with uselessness; drops of it in my eyes blur this moment, this particular jag. Filling up on it, I am sated: there he is, tired and learning to fall asleep on his own, the ray of light bothersome, or the crease in the blanket, the heat, the tear tickling as it brims and falls.

m a y 29

I had read with interest, while still pregnant, about moving the baby to his own crib in his own room. The chapter I'm recalling empathized with the difficult nature of this task, with the mother's anxiety over this separation, and went on to discuss the preferred method for helping baby sleep through the night: letting him cry, alone, and reappearing at ever-lengthening intervals to reassure, until the learned response to his own bed was complete.

I remember reading this section in the book and thinking that the mother who couldn't move her baby to his own room was surely weak-willed. I pictured my baby sleeping happily in his own snug crib, after a few weeks of adjustment to the world. And then.

Then Joseph would cry from his little bedside crib, I'd nurse him with the intention of putting him right back—but we'd both fall asleep. Which was perfectly cozy and convenient for the first three months. But then he began crying every hour. I'd take him in and end up awake all night, afraid I'd roll over on him, afraid Jed would, though he clung to the edge of his side of the bed carefully and willed himself motionless. Joseph was tired. We were tired. The time had come. We moved him out and he cried. And I cried. I wanted him back and happy, which was no longer a possibility. Here was the beginning of unending releases. How to know, with certainty, that he would breathe well on his own, make peace with the dark room, enough to allow his open eyes to adjust to half-shapes and meanderings of light, to find them interesting and not threatening. What would he do without me? And what would I do without him, without the ability to contain his world—watch as it opened and required more of him? Watch him lean into his circumstances, which were positioned, now, at the far end of what once was a very short hall?

)))

This scene is intact: at fifteen, leaving my summer music school and my beloved teachers. Most of them had gone to Oberlin College, and they made, in their radically differing ways, a mosaic of the kind of person I hoped to be; I would go to Oberlin, I decided. Leaving them at the end of the summer, it was obvious that I would miss them; not so obvious was the real reason for the tears: even before the little red house was out of sight, I knew it would always be thus: the leave-taking would never end. Again and again, in one form or another it would occur and there was nothing I could do about it. Not temperamentally inclined, even then, to cling, I knew my present was doing a slow fade, happening and unhappening, even as I held a hand or exchanged an address and promises I intended to keep.

Joseph is four months, and then some. At night I put him down in his crib and he sleeps, more or less, soundly. I am grateful and sit down to work, to read, pulling myself close again, something like buttoning a coat back to neatness, smoothing it over the body's contours after the wind has whipped it around. During the day, loss comes in moments, more patchy than momentous—his wide smile and sure joy at seeing me appear in his doorway after a nap and how, increasingly, that response is interrupted by the distractions of the object world—my hair, watch, earrings—or nothing of mine at all: downstairs, the teakettle's bright expanse, in which he has seen his own altered face.

m a y 3 0

The book that tells about moving baby out is written in a question-answer format. Jed thinks it's patronizing. I said I didn't find it to be so at all. "That's because," a friend said, "as a woman, you're used to being patronized." But that wasn't it; it's more that everything about caring for a child comes, most truly, in the nagging form of a question, trailing its multiple answers behind. Last month, at three A.M., trying to figure out if Joseph needed to be fed or helped back to sleep, or was uncomfortably wet, I (Jed had completed his shift) found myself so stunned at that hour by the possible courses of action, that in order to act at all I had to form an exam-style sequence of responses:

It's three in the morning and your child is crying, relentlessly, aimlessly, in his crib. Should you:

a) pick him up and comfort him
b) give him his pacifier and help him back to sleep
c) feed him
d) take him into your bed just this once

Before I can answer, more questions break in which must be attended; soon they form a branching tree: which of these solutions have I tried already? all of them? well then, in what order and maybe that's wrong? should I simply try them all again, like jiggling a key until the stubborn lock clicks? what were the circumstances under which (a) worked in the past— had I changed his diaper first? fed him just after? And even if (a), (b), (c), or (d) works, perhaps it is working to create a stubborn habit that will soon need to be repeated every night hereafter.

During the day though, my choices and inclinations are intuitive—eat, change, play, walk, sleep, stroll outside—so that when I'm asked outright, "Does he need a diaper?" or "What time did you feed him last?" I'm nearly always at a loss for a precise response. I fed him when he was hungry. He ate what he needed. My continuum is so buried during the day, is such a deep vein from which responses seep up rather than spring whole, fully worded and quantifiable, that it must seem to others I'm thoroughly muddled, inattentive, forgetful.

j u n e 1

Reluctant to feed him his first bit of rice cereal. And terribly excited when he tastes it, likes it, and wants more and more.

j u n e 2

I watch news footage of chaos in Sierra Leone while nursing Joseph. See an old man, hit with the butt of a rifle, stumble, continue to yell and shake his fists at the soldier looting his house. And then I watch them roll over one another, angry and brawling.

Both of these men were born.

Were children.

And strangely down they shrink, in colored pixels, to a jabbering knot.

And whose wise hand shall come to separate them, pulling them, by their tiny collars, apart? How did their disregard grow? How? I am surprised at the stubborn simplicity of this last thought, the stark line it draws between one-dimensional outrage and the tangle of complexity that is violence. And soon, of course, the reasons, the validities for revenge and retribution stretch their shadows across the screen: there comes a voice that holds a scale upon which events are measured and metered, made proportional to the time allotted to tell this story. Then the voice finishes, and the event is again a simple package, lashed with string: the knots upon knots seal closed the event. It is dropped in a dark box and shipped back to nowhere.

Joseph has finished and fallen asleep. I rub his back and carry him to bed. On the way up, I cannot look at the sharp corners of bookcases, the windowsill's dirty, chipped lip, unyielding tiles of the bathroom floor, jutting doorknobs, the hard mechanics of locks.

There is the wide berth I give to the banister point which catches my pockets and how I must feel him firmly in my arms, feel my feet settle heavily on each step in order to move forward at all.

june 4

A week before Joseph arrived, I watched Ann carry Gabriella down the narrow, winding stairs. My breath caught. She was wearing a long skirt and holding her baby with ease, comfortably in her arms, but all I could see was falling. Tiny splints. Breathing tubes. And worse, silence. I was made to say, in a moment, before I could stop it, "Ann, be careful." Ridiculous. She had endured weeks of premature labor, intrusive monitoring devices, and finally, long weeks of watchfulness in the neonatal intensive care unit as Gabriella gained strength enough to come home. I swallowed, made it a warning to myself, walking behind her, unable to see the stairs below me, balancing my weight, going by feel, twisting around the tight bend, the dark passage at the center of the house.

june 5

There are those nights we dream our disasters: Joseph, poised, at the lip of a steep embankment. White water below. A colony of stinging red ants, used like leeches, but swarming the body, going rubbery and curling like shrimp when plucked off. Mud slides. Doors unhinged from the car I must drive to safety. Bad teeth, bad knees crumbling to dust. The green mud of a tornado sky going finally black. Such dreams are counterpoint to the solidity of the time, the bounded and certain physicality of my days; how heavy the lifting of legs up each step, how sweet the honeysuckle tangling over the fence, filling the whole kitchen with its yellowed scent. The sharp prickling of milk letting down. The way the death of one crow called the whole flock to frantic mourning—for a full day they circled the body, lamenting, consoling.

It's been a few weeks now since Ann moved away. I think of her trying to write in her new house in Pennsylvania, alone all day with Gabriella. I think of her touching the things of her life as she walks past, pressing them into her sight--the simplest things: doors, windows, countertops—as she holds her baby girl. She's told me, twice now, about seeing an oriole near her new home. How unlikely its brightness, how it marked the day for her, stepped forth unequivocally as a distinct moment, a foothold, a tiding. I think of her, here, where she used to live, alone at her desk in her prewar row house. The cool bottle green walls, the old milky blue tiles on the bathroom floor. Of how she moved through, with the luxury of distraction, the simple, uncluttered beauty of that place until she was about to leave.

Strangely, I do not wake from the plague and disaster dreams with a sense of urgency, or even anxiety, just the memory of vivid pictures, stills of certain moments: the garnet shine and translucence of one red ant, greatly enlarged, and the sense of having to take care when handling the fragile, impossibly hinged segments of its body. The silty mud of a landslide rubbed between fingers, gritty between molars, drying to a glove of white dust up my arm. The road flying past and the impact of wind as I drive without a door, the rough webbing of the seat belt holding fast. Only a few times since Joseph's birth have I awakened distraught—after dreaming that Jed was leaving us, that he simply didn't love me and could no longer pretend. This dream, of course, at a time when I've seen such joy in his face that he, himself, looks new and bright, surprised at his own laughter. At his own boy. At the unruly shape Joseph and I make of his embrace now.

june 11

How many ways might a day be measured? By the rule of stairs climbed and the weight of groceries hauled up them? By the proportion of dry cereal flakes to milk necessary to make a smooth paste; by the time it takes a glass of cold water to relieve the heat of a long walk? More accurate still is a child's body, that star, that fathom to measure by: plants in the wooded cul-de-sac are knowable by it—a leaf the size of his head, a trunk three Josephs long, or he'd come up to this stalk's first flower, and this bud is as small as his toe, or already as large. And that bird's flight—it loops easily enough for him to track, or, all angle and jab, the starling dips out of his sight and dives too quickly away for him to follow.

The lush, relentless strength of summer fleshes these days, which in their extravagance layer themselves green over green, which in their bounty forget the midst, forget at their center the hard bud of their own beginning.

Singing the old ballad "Who Killed Cock Robin" with Joseph casts us far back—to the dark sleepiness of *then-as-now*, to when the ballad was written, by way of grackles calling outside, angry-sounding as any riotous bird must have seemed—crow or rooster, sparrow even, the admitted killer—working its way into human song and story. And after dinner—a dinner as any might have been, centuries ago, ladled from a single pot, eaten with bread, finished with fruit—the three of us are out again walking. We walk around our block and the next; we walk until Joseph is tired, out of the day and into evening. We walk ourselves a ring and reinscribe it.

The loblollies hold up their stubs of new growth like candles, each branch end with its skirt of green, a shield to catch the dripping wax. Each tree's a candelabrum or a vigil. The new growth is filed sharp at the tip then grows pliable and downy. Quiet hackles. Groomed cockscomb. All six trees are spindly, planted close on the slope to bank the erosion. Ivy chokes the center one and makes it oddly lush, thicker around the middle. Curly-headed. Fringed. An asparagus stalk. A feather duster.

And near this stand of trees, a vine that's tangled itself into a shrub covers the fence; it sends out mild tendrils, a cluster of fireworks held there, exploding with red and mottled blue berries. With the stillness of abundance, or the abundance of rooted things, these bodies accept the hunger of birds and send them out again, filled. Shelters, respites, hosts, hideaways, yes, but these green lives are no humble innkeepers, open at all hours, key under the mat and let yourself in. They are all about their own business.

The loblollies made meager by lack of space, the vines myriad with lack of care. Leaning and thin, buckled and choked, the dead parts hidden, each roots and makes do. Each wants to live in its way, and means to: embellished and fringed. New. Darkly hidden. Inhabited. With a fence buried deep in its heart.

I know the words for conditions and events, however unlikely, that pose a threat to—and here, where I cannot write his name, I will say instead, should any ill wind be gusting through: *What? This little bundle I'm holding? Just apples in sack. A rumor. A wager.*

I know I am not alone in my fears, think of the old practice (Jewish, Italian, Gypsy, and more) of whispering the name of the newborn only to the child, lest the devil hear it and use the name to beguile the baby, to call it away. I read about conditions and sudden events—latent and dormant—and take precautions. I guard against some and fend off others. Check his breath at night on the back of my hand. Sew loose buttons double tight. But I cannot speak of, give voice to the phrases, the acronyms for treacherous sleep and uncertain breathing. If I had to, of course, I would become fluent in the literature of. Read manuals, articles and papers. Use lingo. Converse with experts. But I don't have to. And every day, at some odd moment—tying my shoe, washing a bib, biting into the impossibly tender flesh of a cherry—I feel the luck holding. Even now I'm knocking wood. Even now, I'm surely spitting.

Outside at the far end of our neighbor's fence is a stubborn pile of junk: a tire, a slice of Plexiglass shaped like a shark's fin, a bucket, a trowel thickened over with plaster. The grass grows up around the stuff, and every week the pile gets smaller; it settles in, comfortable with the override, the undertow and tangle. Each week the original shapes pare away further, each thing slips past its definition. That is, I overlook it. Pass without thinking, the jagged edge, the chipping paint. How powerfully the force, meshing over and under, works to conceal its own piecemeal heart. How powerful the drive to build a whole from a randomness of parts—by stillness and sleight, by neglect, by familiarity, in time.

june 18

Tornado warnings earlier this evening. Joseph was quiet as we stepped onto the porch to watch the green sky roll over, to hear the deep inhalations of trees filling with wind. When the sky broke and it began to rain, we moved back inside and stood behind the screen door. Joseph watched birds in their last-minute gatherings land and fly off, swerve and perch. He turned toward the sudden wind chimes at the back of the house. His breathing was slow as the street-trees-house in front of us swayed in the circumscribed square of the doorframe.

Was he frightened? I wondered. I was, and was already planning which archway to run to when the wind raged past. I imagined having to snatch Joseph from sleep and saw us stumbling to the basement as the house blew in on its unattached side, collapsed on the violets in the bay window, the tender aloe, the clock Jed built from found parts.

I thought of Joseph crying then, more from exhaustion after

the heat of the long day, and how he'd come to add the feel of plunging air pressure, the whistle and engine roar of the storm bearing down, to his understanding of the possible, palpable world.

Mine was a worrisome, nagging fear, tamped and alert. I was aware, too, of trying to quell it; aware of the tightness in my singing voice, of forgetting the words to the soothing songs, of pointing out the forms of birds all around us, leaving out descriptions of their nervous preparations, the disruptions in their early evening routines.

What did Joseph come to know of fear this evening? That it is a ringing in the ears, a prickling at the back of the neck? I am not really asking a question here. Fear, for him, is more a response to be tried and decided upon: What shall I do with this? It was present in the first moments of his first bath, where, once submerged, fear and interest commingled, traveled in alternate flashes across his face—what to feel? what to think?—until his temperament, quivering and simple as a compass, asserted itself, and he decided upon a response: Intrigue. Amusement. Acceptance marked by wary regard for the elemental force all around him.

Let fear be for him, for now, a far-off rumbling, the hard *ping* of hail on the sufficient awning. *Outside.* Let him believe my efforts at concealment—framed, foregrounded, and cropped. Let fear pass like the little TV graphic of a storm we watched on the news, a dervish of lines tilted to indicate path and intention. Let it transform, as it does on the screen, to a stamp-sized cloud dropping darts of rain, as the winds settle and pass over and Joseph falls asleep, hot and sticky, arms thrown over his head, the small cage of his chest rising and falling in the nest of my lap, which is sturdily made of two legs at right angles to the unmoving oak floor.

j u n e 21

This gazing at my child is a kind of eating, it is that elementally nourishing. This looking is like green's effect on the eye, relaxing and spreading the rods and cones. The focus and release of a good stretch. That the eye has a sense of its travels, that it journeys out windows, casts over the repetitive spans of bridges, slips past the hair's-width locations of stations on radios, through laden supermarket shelves in search of the blue box, the red can, is a physical truth. The eye's endeavor is an ache and a want. The eye roams and sorts, classifies and knows, too, the far dream of the horizon, that line which isn't a place at all, but an idea about yearning, an idyll, an elsewhere. The eye wedges into a darkness, a small space: sewer or keyhole, the ground left pocked after the fall mums are pulled, the water-dark shoreline pitted by sandcrabs. The eye cinches in, in strong sun like a closed purse, and darts open again in dim light. Its gaze is a muscle in gorgeous use, a hammer finding the nail with one blow. The eye has a feel for hard rock and sweet air, surefooted in shadow, a toehold lifting the whole body up. We say *drinking in*, but the sensation, the collective musculature receiving, is more substantial still. The pleasure of satiety, of *having seen*, is a kind of flowering in the mouth, in the dark cavity of the chest which is where the eye brings the crow's slick, purpled sheen, the pink star of the mountain laurel to rest. How can the eye stand to rest at all, to be shut for hours against the sight of the world? I remember a film I saw when I was pregnant, in which two Italian brothers try to make a go of it as restaurateurs in America. The older brother, the chef, tries to describe his favorite dish to his new love: "It is so good," he says, "so good, that you have to kill yourself after you eat it."

And what of the perfect endings Joseph's face stirs, his whole body elicits? Ending after ending, no ending at all. It goes on— the tasting-and-seeing goes on. More to take in means more for the taking. His eyes, the shape of spoons, or tadpoles resting head to head, his mouth opening so wide in laughter that the sound pops like kernels of corn in hot oil. His smooth, muscled cheeks and brown curls the size of pencil erasers. Jed calls the sensation of looking "internal sunbursts." More a slow-moving pinwheel for me, each full petal tapering to a point, curling like a tongue, then catching up air, each a little cup, a little throat snagging sound before moving toward more and more again. Or it's the slide and turn around a Mœbius strip, this gazing at our son: when the bend and torque of one gaze is complete, another follows, flips over on itself, turns inner to outer and starts again, hiding its beginning, hiding its end, making invisible the moment of renewal.

june 27

After days of oppressive heat and humidity, leaves seem to have regained their form, firmed up their internal scaffolding.

The breeze exchanges sun for shadow and branch for branch, versions of the hand-over-hand game Joseph will soon want to play, again, again, any excuse to collapse in a laughing knot. There's an ease to the sun; the leaves are drawn to it, and even the shade is bolder now, a good, solid dark, weighing the sun's many heart-shaped hands, shouldering them easily away.

Joseph was stuck to me for much of this past week—as he dozed and nursed, as I carried him up- and downstairs and ran errands. There was a spray of dew across his nose and fore-head, his arms and legs clammy, his head giving off heat like a ball left all day in the sunny yard. There were full drops of sweat on his upper lip and in the small of his back, runnels in the folds of his neck and down the backs of his knees.

Blue shows through the trees like water, and trickling, finds a way into the dense blind of green. A bright insistence, it keeps coming on. A blue unmistakable as a red bird in green holly, that shiver and wobble of primary contrasts, the bright bird marked for a larger, fiercer hunger. I mean, a hunger more fierce than the eye's. At the height of this lushness, when nothing is turning, nothing is brown yet, a goldfinch is a blunt ripeness, fat as a lemon and ready to fall. Its brightness is a dangerous beckoning; it is mortally marked. Heavy and slowed by heat, it wafts like a scent and cannot think to fly. It is distracted, as I am, by the plenty.

For months now, this yearning to hold him even as I am there, right beside him, feeding him applesauce, even as he plays with my hands, my bright rings. Even as I lean him against my breast, then prop him upright, in one bent arm, like a package.

In the past young women would plait a snippet of their

lover's hair and enclose it in a locket, the weaving a simple over-under pattern like a tiny blanket, folded perfectly back upon itself. I have such a locket, a gift from my sister. It's a gold heart with a pane of gold bars crossed on either side, the brown mat of some beloved's hair visible inside.

Since Joseph was born, this yearning has formed itself, materialized as a desire for a visible, outward sign of attachment. The bit of his hair that I've cut so far I've been keeping in a silver pillbox.

Years ago, almost every afternoon I'd pass the two shallow rivers below the cliff of cheekbone on the face of the Nigerian umbrella vendor. We both worked outside, as street vendors, in lower Manhattan. Later, there were the three measured furrows on the face of the beautiful student, studying, as I was, in the library late at night. The precisely wrought scars were not evidence of self-disgust, or the bracing pain of punishment; they were not meant to shock or frighten, but to *bind to*. To mark a line, a lineage in.

Scarification. From the Latin: *scarificare*, to record in the senses. To scratch an outline, to sketch lightly. To make an incision in the bark of a tree.

And the sap rises to fill the outline, seeps into the empty place, the gouge that is the beloved's name. And there the name stays for the life of the tree. And the tree bears the mark in its body ever after, even as the trunk thickens and buries the name.

I've always been drawn to the delicate care shown to relics of all kinds: little boxes for splinters and the houses built to hold them; icons gazed upon; rosaries gathered like berries into the palm; bright glass *malocchio* to ward off the evil eye; fetishes locked in velvet boxes; tin *milagros,* tiny arms or legs, bought to pin to the robes of saints; and even statues of the saints themselves, half-human in their itchy woolen robes, their hidden feet, I imagine, floating, perpetually floating inches off the ground.

Once, for a few days, I tried to be Catholic, so I might wear a crucifix. My mother lent her silver-etched confirmation cross, boxed since she was a girl, to the cause. It's a beautiful one, the bottom stave widening out, before whittling to a decorative, tooled point. But ultimately, even then, at twelve, wearing anything made doubt a symbol, rather than faith, as if one couldn't be expected to bear the ineffable quality of faith and instead called on *materia,* heavy in its objecthood, to utter and confirm one's belief.

To know connectedness, then, as an invisible seizing, an arrest, a hidden, perfect stitch. A stitch of pain come on while running. *Pain,* a spade in the soft earth of the flesh: dig here. (*Scar,* from the Greek *eskhara,* "hearth; a mark caused by burning.") *Here,* at the spot animated by heat, pulsing to snare my attention. Attention, a focus beyond all else, into the one and only moment. The moment a presence. And presence a stay against loss unending.

What consecration to his presence in my body? I have no locket with a curl of his hair, no bracelet with an inscription to wear lightly against my pulse.

But just today we were bound together among the multitudes, two in a flood of lilacs, cosmos, sunflowers, zinnias. Our heads, wind-bent toward each other, made the peak of a little tent. The sun was at full height all around us before we left the garden and went home. Before Joseph napped and I was, again, a quiet desert, teeming, moving slowly, banking, conserving the ground of me.

june 28

Alexander Calder drew the profile of a horse with a nautilus-like coil for the cheek and jaw.

A diamond eye.

Corncob teeth.

Top lip and bottom, curled iron handles.

Mane a comb.

A knife-blade ear.

How will the world make a horse for Joseph? How will it come—in changeling clouds and the shattered ice of a puddle? In rivulets on the dusty pane, sliding down long Sunday afternoons? Of course in the wrinkles of sheets, the knotted eyes of pine floors. The frightening eyes of raw planks and beams. Owls there. Dark boots and noses.

It will be, too, in the couch's broad arm, where you rest your head, child, where the split grain is mended and the filler plumps like a noodle, or scar.

It will come in the landscape of the table's underside when you lie down and look up and see the horse leaping, see the horse caught, always caught mid-air, almost over the dark stain under there, the clumsy, smudged star of my fingerprint.

july 4

Sun flares and lights the boxwood at the edge of his stroller, and we've pulled the bonnet down for shade. We are at our friends' old farm for a few days. Joseph is napping in the vigorous breeze with his parents on either side: his east and west are filled by our bodies. In the distraction of heat, sweet air and lengthening shadow, here come the unknowable summer days of my mother as a girl, more alone than ever, after her father's death. Days that must have been as breathy and palpable as this one, clouds huffing along, high in the sharp blue summer sky, the scent of the ocean so near, crass gulls in the center of town calling, and nothing, nothing to do for months until school again. I fashion these details because I do not know in which season he died and do not ask. Not now.

Now is the damp earth after rain, soft and ripe. I believe that when this corn shifts in the breeze, sun is urged into the dark chink where the stalk parts from the ground. I believe that when it sways, it grows, that simultaneously roots sink and tassels reach higher. I believe it is happening before me as I sit and watch.

Before me, but not *before my eyes.*

I do not know, either, my father's days as a boy, though here in the dry garden are stalks the color of gray asphalt on hot Manhattan afternoons; under boughs in the rushing wind is the brief shade of a newsstand and the sound of the el, rattling into a distant station. Here, too, is our common present, in which he builds the impossibly fragile planes, patiently, delicately, with tissue paper bodies, on a board at our kitchen table.

In the maple leaves I looked at yesterday with Joseph, the smallest veiny subdivisions turned and turned again, toward infinitely smaller divisions until they were gone from sight. And after looking so hard, I knew, better than ever, the infinity of unseen moments where I was not. That they were there. Did occur, and go on occurring for my mother, my father, as the leaf in my hand went on occurring.

What I saw next occurred too, though Joseph will not remember it: a father lifted his waking son up in the breeze, so he might grab a small handful of leaves as they brushed past. So the soft green might tickle his head. The iron winch at the barn's peak swung its rope and the swallows went looping out of the black squares of barn doors. Sun hit the boxwood, flaring it, lighting it. Blades of grass, trumpets of bulbs pushed forth. Cornflowers burned their blue naphtha, spilled their green bodies between the two barns. Morning glories crawled over and buried the fence even as the father kissed the boy's head and set him down to crawl off on his own through the soft grass.

july 15

In this tiny garden in England, a stone boy is weathered by rain, his face upturned and worn, his nose a gray pucker. There are shadows for his eyes, an abundant bowl of dark moss on the lap his ruined knees make. And here, at the foot of the brick walk, a spill of clothespins, each with a wire curl for an eye, all twenty or thirty dumped like a catch, a haul piled up, mouths like keyholes, jaws locked in sun. The soft pine of them rubbed dark with use. Shining bodies, tossed and held, wet on the ground, as simply rendered as any Dutch still life. How live they are, and because of them, how lively everything becomes: the lozenges of buttons on the hanging shirts, their whites colloidal; a red wash-basket overturned, the shadows of branches fast wings over it—brilliant barn red, it sits like a throne. Now the clothespins again: scattered bones of a fish in bright sun. Such a harvest: stalks of, sheaves of. Flinty-eyed. And this water-stain bloom on the stone boy, all pooled and blackened; red too, but with the rust of persistence.

)))

In the slant of morning light, the boy's face again, half erased by wind, cheeks flattened, nose a gouge the damp sketched in. Mouth slight and sewn by rain. Lichen splotched across his head, like a hand passing over. It's a face recalled in memory, shaded and uncertain, smoked with atmosphere, worn to its essential planes and slopes. The color of hail. The taste of water from a tin cup. Upturned, which means full of anticipation. Upturned, which has come to mean *give me signs, words for what is happening, for this thing, that thing, what it's called, can I touch it, and why is it, why?*

)))

Early in the afternoon, while nursing in the garden, I turn away from my boy's face to my book. I turn away from Joseph, catch myself doing it, catch myself thinking of the many other chances I'll have to watch him in this way, measuring against the rare moments I find to read these days. But later that afternoon, I will see the calf at its mother, pulling for the milk, and feel a shock of desire. And I know, already the terrible momentum has set in; my body now efficient at producing what is needed, and Joseph at getting what he needs. The sensation of feeding him is as familiar as a necklace warmed to my neck, easily shifting over the ridge of collarbone; it is as familiar, too, as the slow peak of day passing, *four o'clock already*, with its telling slant. It's the sensation of lifting the necklace off, over the head, over each ear and catching the nape's fine hair, that quick wince before putting it carefully away in its box. The neck's slight itch, and the necklace's weight still palpable. The red velvet–lined box. Put away. Soon. Mothers in fields with their young, those mothers with sleek, brown, knobbed, speckled collarbones; those mothers of lambs, mothers of calves, wearing their singular task in the open, wearing the heavy bead of their child. The child's peaked and jeweled face dripping. The facets and clarity refracting. The dazzle of it all pulling down to a dark rest, in the box, in the field of soft grass and of distance.

july 20

Follow the eye up to a mud nest under a gutter, and down again to the hole in the fence for the cat. To the low, sooty roofs of houses across the street, visible from our friends' tiny patch of garden. The squat brick chimneys with simple aerials attached. The cat winding itself around the legs of the chair, settling in the shade of a crescent of greenery. The house martin's white tail balancing at the mouth of the cave that is its nest, at the mouths of the three young ones inside, which are three caves of need themselves. How wild, how loud the whole space is when she returns with food; how quickly she comes to them, how almost immediately she must leave again for more.

)))

Blooms of fuchsia hang down like wet flames, slow drips with waxy yellow centers. Four yellow tears at the heart of each flare. Little hearts that burn for days.

)))

"You're a little brat—get off me now! Get off! Do you want another one?" Walking by. Beyond the fence. In the street, Jessica and her mother. Where is *my* anger now, these days? The slow burns dampen, the flashes of what might have been bright flares dull to runnels of cream. Pink. Oyster gray. New-potato red and velvet apricot—colors without resistance. I cannot bite down without shuddering at their easy give. And the hanging heads of these flowers, a rage of color skirted around. Arms at sides. Tears suspended, buoyed on the cheek of air, caught and pulled. Pleats undone. Smote in green. The hanging heads a *shame,* a scolding shouldered by tractable green leaves.

But this, the mother's hand out there, that imprint is a stinging. A brown tangle of vines bearing young, green thorns. And on Jessica's face, on the other side of the fence, the torrent, the fuchsia, is flushed and growing, is limp with drawing up what little comes from the hard ground where she lives.

july 30

This sparrow next to the dwarf juniper makes the stunted tree oddly proportionate, perfectly bird-sized. But no, up the bird flies and I see the tall oak is more properly constructed to hold the sparrow. So, too, are the thin pines, the arching magnolia which months ago balanced its fragrant pink teacups. Right-sized is a size to be wholly lost in, thoroughly filled by. Earlier, the voice of one cicada, latched to the window screen, filled the room. Like smoke or a fever, sound entered this space, flared and doused itself over and over. I couldn't work. It hurt to sit so close to the hum and siren. I've seen birds wrestle cicadas to the ground, the pure grind of machinery, the music of hunger drawn from them both as they flipped and rolled.

Later, night spread its mottled blanket over the dry grass. Joseph in the wide, white space of the tub is the small live center wanting to see *fill and empty*, that spectacle of renewal, wanting to touch and drink the water more than he wants to sit still and regard, little monarch, the warm eddies up to his chest. And out over the suffering grass gone yellow, the cicadas are back, so many making a heave of sound, their singular voice swelling and receding: water through a funnel circling down fast. Joseph catches threads of water in his hands, grabs at the ribbon of silver poured over his stomach until there's no more. He looks and looks for it, there all around him.

july 31

Andrew Wyeth painted a sitting girl in a yellow dress almost a year to date after his father died. The dress is buttery and she is serene, perfectly poised in the color's warm hand. But more often he painted deer hanging from trees, as if tangled there while jumping, there's that much motion. Deer diving from gray trees to white ground. The thick smoke of the ground inviting the deer down, or surging up to meet them. The dry white of his dog coming in from the winter fields, inhaling deeply, it must be, for there is no breath-cloud at its nose. The red of the barn made metallic in spots by the seep of cold; black pins of ice where the shingles are splitting. What is it about the finest hair, growing over your cheek already: from where does the light resting on it come, so that when I think *snow,* your cheek, even now, midsummer, is a perfect patch of cool?

august 1

The mockingbird in its hail-colored feathers and snowy under-wings, even now in August, is a cool-seeming thing, most heartily itself in the guise of another. Dignified, lovely in its scale and proportion—its elegant neck ever alert to the infinite shapes of danger. Holy jester, never the dandy the gaudy cardinal can be, or earnest as the robin, marked sentinel of simplest tidings. The mockingbird does not solicit the onlooker's gaze, no odd hat, color-shock, characteristic flaw draws the eye; nothing like the one-eared cat that lives nearby, or the jaunty three-legged dalmatian.

Its mocking is nothing at all like scorn, has not a note of cruelty in it. It does not leave off its long apprenticeship for the pleasures of embellishment or exaggeration; just song after song, by the book. Perfect guest and conversationalist, it is all quicksilver and reflection, turned and tuned outward.

It makes beautiful and singular the task of its own erasure.

It is all an aside; its turns of phrase, its phrase-book snippets shift as cannily as currents of air, surprising as earshot, as seeing whatever comes next into range. How borderless it makes the very air; how uncharted again, the disparate strains gathered and twined, bodied in small, gray form.

On Long Island mockingbirds do seagull calls. Here, in their repertoire of up to thirty calls in a row, it is possible to isolate the strains of the Baltimore oriole, that orange shot, once so abundant, as it follows fast from cardinal, to dove, to the simplest brown-toned sparrow. The force with which it sings its acrobatic cadences—surely this is a kind of joy, the spinning out of a song of one's own, fashioned and stitched together from a thrift of air.

Here, then, is the best truth about the instinct for theft: there is no shame in being in love, so in love with a thing you must have it, must use it entirely; there is no shame in being so extravagantly moved that you forget the thing ever belonged to another.

In the open-air market in Warsaw, the hanging pig disappeared daily, precisely, leg by rib by shoulder, until, at the end of the week, the slab of its head alone was for sale. Unhooked from its winch, the head was unbalanced, enormous-seeming without the flensed body, the wings of muscle in the stomach, loosed. Only when it was cheek-down on the butcher's block could I measure rightly: its head the size of my torso. Tip of its pink snout like a balled fist. Pricked ear like a hand raised in greeting. And the gorgeous lashes black and curled, its open eyes blurred milky blue. *In a very deep sleep*. What else could I tell the stunned child beside me?

)))

From the window of a tram when I first arrived in Poland, early fall, a few years ago: what were all those people holding, drumlike in a crooked arm, and picking at as they walked along? And soon I, too, was offered the brown head of a sunflower, dried and bursting with seed, plate-sized and portable. They were sold at every market, stacked on wooden tables like big stuffed envelopes ready to be delivered. Blooms the size of children's faces, each with a stiff, fringed collar at the neck.

)))

Sunflowers: so rightly named, called by their task, to turn toward, and by the act of imitation: how they explode with light before they dip their faces down and dim. My four, on our front stoop, are corralled by their pot, with bristly stems no thicker than an index finger, while our friend Margot's

flowers, staked in her yard, have wrist-sized stalks and blooms
the size of cocked berets, cast-iron skillets, hubcaps spinning
along a straight, easy road.

)))

Here, in the fish store, the perfect bodies of shad and flounder,
salmon and trout are laid out on ice, their flash stilled, eyes
refracting greens and purples, mouths wide in the killing air.
Here are their saw-teeth, needle-teeth, pink gums for sucking;
hinged and wrinkled mouths parted in translucent silence.
They are beautiful to look at, but it's the proximity that really
stuns: the slips of their bodies once at a safe distance, bending
through depths as easily as light rays, their masses of movement that together meant *shadow*, here now. They lived
contained in that watery dimension until they were hauled
into the strata of our gaze. Which makes them ours. Sharp
gills, spiny crenellated backs, teeth for gashing, pliable little
scythes of scales; purpled squid; pale hooks and commas of
shrimp; jellyfish in the Chinese market, a bed of dimmed,
blown peonies—all for us. The striped bass, called rockfish
here, renamed for what it moves around, what it has grown to
resemble. And how we've named the trout *rainbow*, the child's
word for all we know of light's heady transformation in air.

august 8

I've lost something. Mislaid it. Put it in a place that is *away* and
not here. Put it somewhere and I can't remember—but I *do*
remember, walking through the house, through the quiet—

what it looks like, what it means. Earlier, I let it go and now I
cannot hold it. How I miss it. Surely it knows just where it is
and *I'm* the lost thing, really. Words fashion a line to it, bind,
combine, configure space so that, lost as I am, I might sniff
along the breeze, retrace the path thought made.

Joseph is gone, for the first time, to his babysitter. So what
will mark me present now, what mark me with his presence?
Here is the soft rug where he rests his head for a moment
before trying to crawl again, and here, a basket of colored
rings. There are his books and a felt ladybug. Red Chinese
slippers hang on the crib's rail—he likes to swat at their little
cat-faces. The quiet along every wall is the absence of his rising
voice. How the very air has flattened out.

Without strategy, without the hem of hours around me,
I start this unbounded bit of morning, this sitting down to
work, by watching the black-and-white head of the woodpecker chip bark from the pine and stutter its way into the soft
hidden part. Descend the dark length of the trunk on one side.
Fly up to start again on the other.

a u g u s t 11

My hand on the table on the rough grain. The knuckles cut
where I grazed the doorjamb entering with packages. The dirty
windowsill and its collection of paint chips, loose caulk, the
dead wasps fallen from the nest the man from the phone
company sprayed this morning so he could reach the cables to
splice in. He carries the poison with him and as a matter of

course takes down bees' nests, the paper cities of wasps, those mud and spittle globes smartly tucked in eaves and rafters, deep in protected joists. And there the wasps live by the hundreds. There they live by the decisions of their bodies: build here. Stay. Make a path to these bushes and back. Relay dimensions of the world to others, good chinks to turn into, updrafts to ride. And here is danger to mark and veer from, a larger, still hungrier thing than we are. And then a cloud settled on the whole of their work, the very scent of it a panic that swelled their bodies then seized the thread, the wire-fine filament that was a central nerve. The bodies have dropped to the steps below, commands gone out of them, wings stopped midflight, the black lace and fine mesh stiffening.

We bought the spring-loaded traps and set them out. We built and painted a shelf for the phone, high up, and tacked loose wires to the moulding. We dismantled the stereo and moved it into a heavy pine cabinet with sliding doors and stuck a dowel in the track to lock them shut. Rolled and stored the rough hemp mat and bought a fleecy cream-colored rug, speckled with browns like a patch of marsh land. The unused sockets are plugged and cabinet locks installed in the kitchen. We bought new traps and set them out and caught three mice immediately.

"So—your life must have changed completely," an acquaintance comments at the farmers' market. It's part question, part assertion. It's Saturday morning. I have piled the loose potatoes around Joseph in the stroller after the bag split, and I'm heading for the car. He holds a small red potato in each hand.

He pats them, bangs them together, digs his nails in as I try to angle the bright sun out of his eyes, keep more potatoes from falling, sign the petition to save the local library, keep his waving arms out of people's bags, his face from hitting the rail of the stroller—he is chewing on it—as we go over bumps. The strawberries out of reach. The keys, pulled from my knapsack, from poking him in the eye as he shakes them to make the sound go, the light catch.

But she means "Are you up all night? Can you work? Are you exhausted?" She means "Can I do this too?" She is listening to herself listen to my words, sifting for new desire, or knowledge to weigh against her own uncertainty.

Forms of plague are carried by rodents, in their urine, in their feces. Mice are host to ticks and fleas. Joseph's nearly crawling. They eat our fruit, leave droppings in our silverware drawer, in pots and on the stove. Around the breadbox. Along the baseboards.

I am driven to expedience by motherhood, as I was to patience by pregnancy.

She is looking hard at me as I answer, but nowhere do the dizzying contradictions show.

august 12

When Ann was moving and there came a morning that was the last morning I'd see her in Baltimore, there was a long moment, minutes really, in which we held on to one another, and pressed belly to belly there in the street, came to know something we might never have allowed had we not both so recently had children.

The comfort passing between, the passed-beyond-words of that moment was not the bodily comfort of familiarity, casual in its dailiness: shared clothes or drinks or a kiss hello. Certainly, it was a stay against circumstance, against being taken from each other, but too, it was a moment enacted in newly acquired mothers' gestures: with arms that held our babies to feed and lifted them away again, satisfied; with slumped bodies, half dizzy with the exhaustion of soothing children late at night. There, in the street, the door of my car wide open, the habitual rocking was stilled—that paced, synchronized swaying we mirrored in one another, standing together, hushing our babies—completely stilled, so that we might move more singularly together, ourselves pulled by the rhythms of solace and full in our sadness.

And again, with Patty this summer, dear friend whom I hadn't seen in years, there it was: the two of us saying goodbye at the airport, then turning back to our husbands and our boys, away from the body of another woman, replica of one's own, loosed, unveiled, and held. Patty's tall elegance, and Ann's small, contained grace. Hipbones, once again, prominent points to lean into. The scent of their hair, the hands I'd seen so many times before—at rest, around mugs and the stems of wine glasses, floury, dirty, unstudied on their child's body. Turning pages. Moving over their own written words. I remember how I touched Ann's hair before she turned to leave. I hadn't meant to; it seemed an almost brazen assertion of motherhood, a move so filled and fraught with tenderness— and how often had I winced at the kindness shown me, frantic not to be hemmed by my own mother's consolation, impatient with my own need for it. But there was also a hand on my shoulder, my neck touched, my own head close against a shoulder, resting there, the full weight of it held firmly, dependably up.

I thought of those movies in which the plane is about to go down, the sky a tilting, broken blue out the small porthole, the swell of music rushing toward doom. And the protagonists, the near-lovers—under pressure of all that will be lost, and the heft of finality—kiss. Passionately. With relief and longing. And in an awkward—for the plane is shaking—culminating act of truth, all the long-withheld complexities are released.

And what of this desire between women, the drive to be physically present to one another, bodily known—not sexually, which would be both to freight and to simplify the power of this expression—but certainly passionately. I mean, with knowledge of an end apparent; the end of walking and reading, eating and sitting together; of our astonishing and meager physical selves together, but for a few times a year. And so, gone mother to mother like that, the body I returned to was charged and stirring—with absence, with presence—and in those too-quick, parting moments, came to know something of what the shape of myself as *mother* feels like.

august 15

At the art museum's cafe today I sipped an iced coffee while Joseph nursed. We sat outside near the fountain at a table fitted with a simple white umbrella; it was like sitting under a stretching canvas. Sparrows were washing in the crevices of wet stone at the fountain's edge; some near our table were pecking at a bread crust. On the slate beneath my feet were scattered metallic confetti from a party—little cutouts in red, gold and blue. They fell between the stones' cracks and flashed where they caught in the azaleas, bloomed months ago. *GO GO GO* I thought they read at first, an urgent message, here, as I had just settled down. Then *60,* I realized. *Impossible,* I was thinking. Not impossibly old, but impossible to know now, in the same way I cannot accurately feel *winter* when the surge of wings and weak breeze fills this courtyard, cannot sense the dissolve of individual forms under white, limbs gone ochre, then downy silver, where now lush green collects. In winter the window in my room will be relentlessly drafty, my hands tight around the pen, breath condensing on the pane, the early dark turning it to a mirror as I sit to work.

Today is my mother's birthday. She's sixty-three. I could not imagine having a child as near as a few years ago, could not fit the shape of my mind to this unknown rhythm, this person, this face. Now, as we have him with us daily, so the desire grows, to be more and more similarly upended, to be taken up by the collar and swung senseless into what I cannot know; to be proved wrong, or to have the merest leanings, wordless and unacknowledged as they are, proved right by leaps of faith. To be tricked out and felled; to fall and roll far.

A young woman sat down near us, near the fountain in the shade of the big oak. She ordered tea, and it came in its own creamy pot, with a bright steel strainer and a pink napkin. She was lovely—a short cap of black hair, square, thin shoulders leaning over the cup, the steam a plume the wind carried away from her lips. But best was the way she read, with a mild, changing expression on her face, looking up and out beyond us, considering a passage or sentence or word. I've done the same, absorbed by the internal pace a book offers—in cafés in other cities, other countries, and here, too, in this same place, before Joseph.

And she smiled at the sparrows tumbling over one another, contained in her own person; how contemplative, how amused I imagined her to be. Spare in her black dress and black sandals. And what was she reading? Italo Calvino's *Invisible Cities*—fables of cities-as-women, each memorable in its singularity? Anything at all by Pablo Neruda, who said, "It is good, at certain hours of the day and night, to look closely at the world of objects at rest." Mary Oliver, who, at the end of her poem "The Summer Day," asks for us all,

> Tell me, what is it you plan to do
> with your one wild and precious life?

She sipped her tea, brought a finger to the corner of her mouth, her hand curved as elegantly as a dancer's, infused with the whole quiet energy of the body and composed in its grace. She tipped the book up—the latest, I imagine, all raised silver and hot pink, a hardback, I could see, by Sidney Sheldon.

august 18

Early this morning the tree cutters came to the lot out back. All morning they labored. And when the work began, I welcomed the sounds of saws and motors, the whine in the background, the template of plot laid roughly over the morning. It was the axis rotating the world made audible. Things and people set in motion and staying so: accounted for, busy, useful. It was improvement under way, a thinning out around the power lines, which spark so frighteningly in strong wind, a trimming of limbs, fallen while we were gone this weekend and storms passed through. This was the noise of the world at work, the constituting rumble of good decisions, of order convening and sensible forms reclaimed. Voices were calling, words plowed under or stobbed by the rise and turn of grinding machines, the rake of metal on metal.

I look up to see whole trees coming down, the sky biting deeper into the stand of pine, oak, and locust. The sky, once a slow blue drip into green, is now a cascade falling farther, faster down.

Now the men's fractured voices seam up into words for places and procedures, into short snaps of laughter. Accented directions. The sickly crack-crack as they push down the notched trunks, the sound of a tooth moving in its socket, the sound of bone conducting vibration. The awful twisting-and-thudding, by late afternoon, is no longer sensible, well-intentioned white noise, no longer anything to absorb and layer over my own work. The sulky power broods and bears down. The sound is pitched at the heat of commerce: force and resistance, the drive to completion playing out before us. Unfurling like a banner. Unleashed and snapping.

Joseph wakes from a nap, disoriented; sleep's blank geography fills too quickly with the loud, waking world, the odd masses of shapes in his room: hunched dresser, white crooked arm of the mobile which holds flying pig, donkey, tiger. I pick him up, walk slowly through the house reacclimating as we go: *Here, in the quilt, is the star and the flower; here you are, that's your face in the mirror. Here's the bird's eye, the book, and the table.* And then, when we've walked through the whole quiet house, we go outside to watch the clearing, the erasure of the bounded lot, the sky come falling toward us.

august 19

Joseph and I visit the miniature displays at the museum—colonial New England scenes behind panels of glass, eye-level for him, riding in his pack, facing forward. He claps and squeals at the wooden clock, numbers the size of quotation marks; a dappling through one set of panes suggests sun-in-the-orchard, and in the next scene, a brooding, green glow is the stormy sea past the windows of the captain's bedroom. Chairs finely upholstered, bright slivers of knife, fork, and spoon on the table. On a bed a stuffed bear the size of a fingernail. Eyelash fringe on the eyelet curtains. Painted meniscus of wine in a glass and a thimble-sized tureen of soup, orange spots for carrots, white for potatoes. Joseph's hand the size of a rocking chair, a captain's chest, a portrait of an ancestor looking sternly down. And then, when this all satisfies and room after tiny lit room has been shown, we go off to the contemporary wing. Up the marble stairs, through the magenta, blood orange Matisse shapes: the steady cup on a tilting table, pinned there by its own quiet yellow force, by the unmistakable health of the pink hand moving, perpetually, toward it: how the tea waits under its coil of steam and the full cup is an oasis come upon in the wilds of curtain, coverlet, painted painting.

We move past the buffed Mœbius strip of marble, rose marble, egg-speckled, so shiny and—*No, don't touch*, the guard says to Joseph, whose hand is already patting the cool, thick curve where I've let him roam.

And there, before us as we enter, must enter, through the beckoning arch, is the pink horse. I say "See how big!" to Joseph. And he looks, but the pink horse is really two horses, *Dos Equis*, by Susan Rothenberg, one an erasure, a shadow of the other. Horse and protohorse, I'm thinking, the second thought curving over, remaking the first . . .

But Joseph spreads his arms and kicks at the expanse of color. He follows my finger tracing in air the horse's ear, the size of his forearm, the horse's head, double the length of his body. We find the sharp anvil of the front hoof, and up we ride the taut curve of the fetlock; all around the rump his eye goes, then back under the crescent of dipping belly, while I feel the movement in his neck, in his turning body, and in his arms that, stretched as wide as they go, hold the horse, both horses, close.

august 26

Driving past a playground, I see a girl standing in the middle of a group of younger children; she is holding, no, pulling one of them up by the collar, shaking the collar, and the little one is standing on her toes to slacken the grip on her shirt, to ease the tension. Such a quick take—had I sneezed I'd have missed it—of how even the smallest bodies assume the forms of power and capitulation. How already they know the postures of force—the terrible raised arm, the arm drawn back through which anger flashes, which is a lightning rod for it. How the smallest body adapts to anger, becomes suddenly less, assumes a bent pose, which in its terrible compliance induces greater wrath still. The big girl is a revelation herself, an entire household in a frame, its tenor, its terror, the gestures well learned and reproduced here, to mitigate her own smallness.

)))

The cicadas' hum is a tearing of fabric. A fast rip of stitches, an entire dress-length. The amplified pour through the cinched waist of an hourglass. Shards over which the whole day is pulled toward its end.

)))

In the grocery store I saw a baby, maybe ten months old and so heavy, so bloated that he was propped straight by his girth and could not turn side to side or bend forward in the cart. And when he smiled, only his lips moved; there was no room at all for his thick cheeks to dimple or pouch, so terribly puffed were they. The whole of him was piled around the core of his buried spine, a mass of soft yarn badly raveled and slipping from its spool, collecting in a rumple. The lovely flax of his hair, the shells of teeth in his wet mouth were difficult to find, to rest the eye on. The bulk of him was a curiosity, and I was aware of my looking as a kind of cruelty as it revealed and rested on his helplessness. To his tired, heavy mother, just ahead of me on the check-out line, I said, "He has such beautiful eyes." And he did. They were violets. And with them, the child watched me watching him, hardly able to look past his body, my pity the weight of a heavy shawl he shouldered, even then, in the warm store, at the end of August.

august 30

He holds his fist up and turns it over in the pour of light, in the dust motes of the clear, first rays through the living room's bay window. He turns his hand royally or as if unscrewing a light bulb, watches the mesh of fingers stop when he holds them high, start when he wants them to move again, according to his command; the funniest thing in the world to him, and he laughs at his willing hands in the sun, at the whole trick of fulfillment.

)))

The heavy one suffering in the heat; the dog gone wild at the end of its short chain; young women I teach who are afraid to eat, of what more they might want if once they were filled; the ugly, orthotic shoes at the cobbler's shop and who would come for them and how; the woman on the street wearing too much makeup, and the frightened look of someone left with only herself to convince; an old man carrying a bag of vegetables walking home from the farmers' market, holding the heavy package on the bottom and stopping every few steps to rest, I mean, the flaw—slight or glimpsed as it is in anyone—is more distinctly arrayed these last, fiercely bright days before fall.

Gashes in a tree trunk where the sap welled and slicked over, where a car jumped the curb and tore the silvered skin ragged.

In the woods, on hard quills of pine needles, the way an aluminum can, crushed compact-size, holds its saucer of gaudy light.

)))

What would have come next, here, in this spiral of thought, in this space, had Joseph not woken and called me away? Here, where I stop, stray notions about fulfillment, about frailty, a barrage of it, are tethered somehow, if not yet by the muscle of thought well flexed, then by a stubborn exposed sinew of it, pulled taut between, thin as a file, a strand of hair. A light bulb's filament, that coiled snap, waiting.

september 1

Joseph became, in her arms, the infant she held nearly twenty years ago. And in hers, the child she never had. In yet another's, her own boy, small as he was just scant months ago. Passing my own son around the gathering of women, I watch him in their embraces, some mothers, others not, most older than I. He becomes a recollection, a body's memory, as he rests his head on a shoulder, as he is expertly propped in a bent, sturdy arm. He becomes desire intensifying. And the object of desire, fulfilled years ago. I see him amidst the wire rims of glasses, keys held out, their cold music loosed, his *oh-oh-oh* of delight as he is passed from embrace to embrace.

How is it then, that this child stirs such a willing blur of boundaries, and the child in the public bathroom, spanked and shaken for not washing her hands properly, would not, could not become this one's child, that one's child. Was, that day, no one's desire. And neither was she mine. For we all remained silent.

And neither was she mine.

I had not made her mine.

Not yet.

For that happened nearly six years ago, before I could imagine myself a mother. I did not say a thing. Today she would be my ten-year-old girl; in ten more years, my recollection, as Joseph is, now, their recollection.

My own baby.

She must have been four then.

I remember her face, as any mother recalls, too clearly, the face of her lost child.

september 6

I'd think of the fuss, what seemed then, before Joseph, to be such excess on the part of new parents: their endless devotions, their careful tending, all primping and patting. I'd balance the extravagance I saw by conjuring a myth of strength and sense—that primitive, bearing her child alone, in a field; squatting, releasing it into the day, the same day that would take her back to her work, to the laden fields, because she was able, after a rest, and because circumstance required it. Birth would hardly break the cadence of her day. I admired her and her sorrow too; rather, the way she'd muscle down sorrow, muscle the child into a wrap knotted over her breast where it would stay, in the scurry and drone of her life, another demand met.

This must be the same mythologized figure, who, years hence, old and failing, would set off alone for ice floe or dark wood to take herself cleanly out of this world? I thought of her competence, discipline, rigor. Cumbered by nothing, she'd walk through the day with her child, the same way she'd walk out of her life. Directly, with no fuss. Not the fuss of new parents I knew, so expressive and constant. "Precious," I'd think, meaning lacking a natural grace for the mundane—the diapering, feeding, checking for fever. Sentimental even, a kind of damage done to the present and real in the name of an idealized past. How disproportionate they seemed in their hovering, so far from her way, from the way wild things lay down with their young, give over their bodies entirely, then nudge the children away when ready to rise and move on. Good instinct—the lion's, the dog's—I imagined, came without frill. No "open up for the plane—here come your nice peas."

But now.

Now I want sound, cadence, and rhythm to fill the ear richly; I want slower unfoldings and unalloyed shifts; to know more still of others' contentious, failing, stubborn belief, their wranglings written down the long (or dense, or deft, or perfectly spare) body of the poem. Now the poem's seams can split, tear, unravel. Now my own responses fleece over, petal up when I see his face. My responses vault, billow, and trail; are not snapped open like a shade or watchful eye on duty, all readied nerve and resolve. The time I have, I take to look at him. To watch, which is to be struck, clear-cut, swept, and reseeded. I need not move toward any task, at that moment, past gazing on the face of my child. Joseph's face, his hand in thrall, turned to the shadow of a branch on his body, late afternoon, presents itself in place of task, and no daily distraction, no practical reason takes me from it.

Joseph's face, his hand in thrall, cannot be weighed; they weigh nothing at all. They crash to earth, clatter and rock. Correspondence, the pile of dishes, the phone loudly ringing, shake and fly from the epicenter at the moment of impact: this spot of sun on the polished floor. This sticky spoon, this caned rocker, unweaving.

Awe is not precious; it looks to be spent, to be shot away whole, that it might renew. It is nothing the woman in the field can spare, all matter-of-fact attention-paid as she is, voice and food given when needed, yes, but her awe overrun with work and worry. And that strong, calm competence of hers I so admired, the clean lines of efficiency and the grace of diligence, are sad and poor beside the petting and the adoration. Her time is meager beside the time we can lose, overspend, and still draw on, pulling curls, biting ears, doing nothing but pointing out *tree, car, dog*—these moments which, by anyone's standard, constitute truest luxury: that which one has fast grown accustomed to and cannot, will not do without.

september 7

And he who stocked the meat, who laid the wrapped loin,
chop—*haunch* it was when once it lived—down in the cool
refrigerated bed, watched as they passed. He held a tray of
fresh-cut parts and watched the boy follow close to his father,
and quickly. He watched the father's words cut in, saw how
they landed on the boy's thin frame, though the boy was
almost as tall as his father, saw the father cut his way through
the crowd and the son follow in the narrow space left open.
And the packer stood there with a full tray, watching, way past
the point at which the father's words could be heard, the cold
tray heavy, the apron he wore reddened, and the gloves and hat
too, straight from the big freezer he worked in. And the father's
shoulders, so thick under his blue shirt, how they angled like
paddles through the crowd, and the boy's, like blades, two
sharp crescents, were incomplete as a sketch: the boy was
sketched there in the store like an animal running the length of
a cave, Lascaux or Dordogne, pulling its flat body along,
darkened by the eclipse of a bear, the bear darkened by a
mountain, that mountain slumped in the shadow of another
more looming still, the whole sequence caught in the eye of
one who thought to pause and see it all.

september 13

Perfectly, cruelly, the sunflower jackknifed in heavy rain. The
stalk of its spine snapped under the pelting. The cement walk

to our house began to lift from its bed, floated up from its solid hold, broke from the mainland, and moved in chunks toward the street. The drain, a hell for the smallest of us: beetles and spiders with ingles in their bodies for holding air, skeletons as delicate as the dry spines of leaves, overcome by the filthy waves.

While I was at school, the cars collided. Each of my students was nearing the classroom. The paths they cut were spokes toward the brief center we'd make together for fifty minutes. And then paths turning back to construct further webs of intention, indecision, and whim.

While I was at school the cars collided; my husband and son inside our small red one, whole, but the very door I had locked and patted goodbye crushed shut. Then every random thing was stilled and flush with consequence. Slowly the stranger— the woman, whose car would have safely passed Jed's had the stop sign been cleared of a low, broken branch—became a name; three names, an address; then customer of a company that would pay for the condition of her fate that morning. And after minutes of standing, breathless, in front of her smashed car, in front of her silence, the longer we stood in the wash of spinning lights, the more likely it all seemed. The day's fret-work visible, its scaffolding grown sturdy.

While I was at school my husband was thinking—nothing really, at that moment. My son was playing with his stuffed orange tiger when our paths were made to loop back upon each other's, odd unseen paths, colors as benign as the New York City subway map's, the pinks, greens, and yellows tying the down-below dark trenches together. Veins are plotted blue and red in anatomy books. Warp and woof are channels of repair in the world of the loom, a simple maker of solidity; *go over and under* it says and says. And the clicking of the shuttle moves toward and away, toward and away, no violent gesture snags the eye from its rhythm. Just every few rows, stop and observe, comb the lines tight and the fabric holds.

While I was in school, about to move from office to class and trail the thread of my own plot behind me, slipknot it with his, with hers that day, with the infinite, unknowable stories of others, I was called back to see the design, the lit shape of the design thick with incident: the uneven banking of the car's path over the curb and my son and my husband afterwards, upright, unbent, amidst the buckled and thrown parts. There we were, in the lightest rain, in the spinning red lights, the yellow, the silver broken bits shattering the street's gray tedium, thrown stitches of the Navajo weavers, those mindful, plotted imperfections added in to appease the spirits, to deny any inclination toward perfection. The crows on power lines. Our tracks sketched in mud, the noise of the accident already a bright sliver in the minds of the birds lifting off. Looking up, I saw them pass over us, trailing their own invisible ribbons, flying ahead over the paths we, there below, were already redrawing.

september 18

The sunlight in runnels this morning off the magnolia, the same light-through-dark pour as waves breaking on the jetty *at home* I still say. Long, thin branches of the crape myrtle dip and bob their gathered blossoms, like the strung pods of seaweed worked into motion by currents and tides. "We're going home to see my parents," I'll say to a friend, and Jed asks later, "Isn't *this* your home?" Of course it is. In fact, so much is this now my home that the thought of leaving fills me with dread. Yes, friends are here, and the paths to doctors, and I know where to get beveled washers for the old sink, who runs the quickest dry cleaners, and that best I like the new Russian cobbler a few blocks away, not the surly one in the shopping center, though others I know swear by his work. I imagine myself in another state, in another part of the country, say Arizona, teaching there, without the Cylburn Arboretum to wander after classes. Without, any time I want it, the old mansion at the heart of its leafy grounds, just past the white garden and the pink garden, its small, educational nature room with turtles in formaldehyde, dried starfish, and musty, stuffed birds with broken beaks badly glued. Long, low wooden tables the children sit at and turn over in their hands—my child, in his hands—the skeleton of a squirrel, crabs' claws, the black hood of a plushed milkweed pod, its downy seed bed gray and rumpled after seasons of use.

)))

I have never known what to make of the Paulownia's huge heart-shaped leaves, unlikely-seeming and tropical-looking as a neighbor's outdoor cactus bed, lost things claiming their place by force of will, whose best latitudes seem many degrees from here, their most comfortable homes wetter or drier, more ferocious, at least more theatrical.

)))

The song of the gas man, come to read our meter. The clipped end of the word *man* as his voice rises, and the word is drawn and doubled in length: *May-in!* Hearing the tune come closer. House by house, waiting. Not opening the door until it rings with his song.

)))

"A-rabers"—Baltimore's traveling produce vendors. Ours, one of a handful left, with his horse pulling the cart of fresh fruit and vegetables down our street, early evenings in the summer. The small old horse and the small old man. The horse's bridle decorated with plastic flowers, red ribbons, the cart looking parade-ready, with fringes, tassels, and bells, going under the trees, past all the simple houses. People running out with their money.

)))

The red fox. Squalls of winter storms sealed us in, sealed the raccoon and opossum, the reservoir's carp and bluegill, deeply in their darks. But the cold pushed the fox to our front stoop, one afternoon, two years ago now. I opened the front door for no reason at all and there saw the feather of its body, the burnished blade of its tail arc past, and slip away into the woods. The snow was packing up hard, but the fox hung over it like smoke and never broke the surface, just scratched a few claw marks in. Like any bird would, finding its footing, before it flew up and was gone.

)))

We thought we were making a place for a child, moving desks, clearing books to make a room for him. Boxing up. Setting high on shelves. Wrapping and storing, among so many things, the little relic Jed found in Israel when he was a boy. That finger of opaque blue glass. I've always been a little wary of it, unsettled, until I picked it up and really looked: it's a *spout*, pocked and scratched. Roman glass—fragment of another place entirely. And from a smaller geography still: a kitchen. Hot water through it, or clear, cold milk, tinted blue. Or wine. Or it was a child's plaything, small as the spout is, and he watered his seedlings with it. That was his job. This child who has come to fill our kitchen with his voice, who fills our time from his generous cup, fragile cup from which hours pour.

september 29

Open as a palm in asking, a sack wide open, sack of grain, sack of sugar, so terribly soft were the white bellies of the mice. In the position of sleep, caught in a place where the body unspools its memory of the interior. Open as fear, their forms stock as slapstick, limbs at all angles feeling for footholds, for solid ground in their terrible falling.

How spare the two bodies on the stove's white enamel. How filled they looked, yet not unnaturally, with gases collecting, with the systems' stoppage. How features at the end look, too, like reviving, held breath or near-singing, a body in the process of drawing sweet air. How lively the deer looked in the yard we passed; it was hanging, yes, from a tree, and flying it seemed or diving back down, a body captured in the poise of intention.

And also in the yard, the shot raccoon, its skin tacked high on the barn's east wall, the compass of its head tilted northeast or just up, nose to the wind, craving some wilder scent it caught there.

And though they were dead, they were not ever-luckless cartoon animals, the underdog crashed into a wall, jaw and body one single plane, flat as a frying pan and falling away from the stylized brick wall, shut door, black Acme safe, poor chump who goes spinning and clattering down like a penny to rest.

I set more traps before we left. It was the last thing I did before closing the door. I put four out and dabbed the under-side of each coiled spring with thick peanut butter. So the mice would have to work to get at it and thus by their own desire and effort be caught. I thought it all through. I considered the sequence and dimensions of plot, how it would start, the play of events. And when we came back to the overturned bodies, I expected them. And it wasn't without satisfaction that I found the first and then the second and thought, with the weight of the trap half-covering their bodies, how overcome they looked. The balsa-wood trap like an operating room sheet draped to isolate the work site.

So here I will go to work on their bodies, here, on this page drape, then reveal, as I can, the slackness they became. I will clear a new space for the sight of them. Here, in their death, I will give the dark loam of these moments, this time, give my conjuring will, and as explanation, my drive to keep my own young one safe, clean, because—forgive me—I threw the mice away. Because I did not bury them. Because I did not set them

under a smooth stone or find a box or cover them with the
puzzle-shaped leaves of the maple, as I imagine Joseph will
want to do in a few years' time.

october 15

I'm seeing it now with Joseph, close up: the lip of the blue
watering can, sharp where the plastic leaked and was cut from
the mold, sharp where the seam of the handle sealed up in a
ragged pinch. And in the white junction box along the base-
board, a small hole at the top the width of a finger and the only
finger to measure by, his. I'm down here now, face to the floor,
to see whirlygigs blow in through the front door, to see, days
later, how they've dried to brown wings and crumbled to
sharp-edged dust. Later, outside, the fence slats halve and half
hide my face; they stripe out one eye, then another, in quick
switches. Then they are ribs that sound thoroughly hollow, so
satisfying to run a stick over, so painless to poke a stick
through.

)))

His hand on the mesh of his playpen and mine pressing back,
the honeycombs making pockets of flesh, little flesh-pocks,
fish-in-nets we tease and make jump, finger to finger. *Gentle* I
say as he grabs the dog's skin, loose at the neck, opens and
closes small handfuls until she turns and licks him away. And
hear the event of notes interrupted on the piano, as he picks
from a cluster of tones just one, and plays it over and over, a
steady voice rising, bright descant over the brooding colors the
left hand is finding and stirring.

)))

Balls of wool pulled from the carpet have a dense center, an outer corona thinning to breath, a nimble-spoked haze that turns over in the gust and wake of footfalls.

)))

Monarchs unhinge themselves from the red maple, from dry stalks of the last tomatoes, pump their wings, which seem heavier this month, then lift into the air, stitch and bob, slip and gather, and the eye can't catch all the quick decisions.

)))

New blue curtains the color of jays, and this morning, the surprise of them hanging there as—*no, don't pull*—the sun presses in, the wind—*no no*—fills the pleats all the way to the top where the white rod is run through. See? Wind *blows* and the curtain comes close; you hide your face and the light goes away, and the cars and I go, until you put us all back again with your looking.

)))

Fat pumpkins press against the bars of their body, thick ribs near bursting as they grow, tethered and tangled in the field. They are ready to be pulled from the vine when, tapped, they make the sound of small steps. The sound of small steps we, now, can imagine.

)))

From a small, green cup, bath water pours out in a silver scarf, a magic scarf that breaks into bits on the surface of itself and disappears. Rinse water lifts his fine hair in a wave like sea grass that clings to the jetty's boulders and rolls out with the tide, then settles over the outcrops of ears, the soft fontanel, that imprint in sand, already disappearing.

)))

Then there's the feel of the pages of books, the black ciphers
linking across and across in neat rows until the whole field is
laid down and the eye walks along each station of thought.
Such an urge, I know, to pick the words up, to scratch them off
the white page, to pry then to press the dark rim of them under
a thumbnail. How the code means, every time, the same
sounds from the mouth, and the mouth any mouth; it's the
repetition that's holy. My mouth, the black signs, and the
little girl dressing, the little girl eating, *banana* she loves,
the breathing increases, recognition, *toothbrush*, increases,
pajamas, the shout comes, the chant, tune and refrain: these
words are the *world*.

october 16

I am walking down the stairs in the middle of the morning
after Joseph has gone for his nap, after the usual routine:
fussing, standing, babbling *mamamama* until I lay him down
and down again, pat his back, say, "It's time for a rest." I am
going down and I am thinking of quiet, yet a voice is sounding.

I place and release my steps in careful measure on the
sturdiest parts of the floor—step too lightly and the slow
pressure sustains the sound, like a mint unwrapped painstak-
ingly at a concert. I have learned the positions of quiet by now,
keen as stencils of feet on a dance studio floor, and descending,
shift toward the thick lip of each stair. Those spots are less
vocal than the throaty centers, bearing direct weight for the

fifty or so years of this house's life. Still, the creaks underfoot are pitched at the level of his waking cry, and so, in this way, the climb down is always full-voiced, even when Joseph is out for a walk with his father or sleeping soundly.

When Joseph is out for a walk with his father and I am at home, the house is pained and alert. I step and cringe: it's the same powerful sense of transgression I felt as a child, when *step on a crack, break your mother's back* was unleashed, and I worried over the incident my misstep would cause. By now, when he sleeps, the noisy stairs, the swollen hinges, even the window that drops unexpectedly down do not startle him anymore.

But at dinner he turns to our phone when he hears a ringing in the house next door and wonders, looking from Jed, to me, to the phone again, "Why don't they pick it up?" He points and urges. And I talk and explain, in the face of my own wondering at how the breaking of pattern itself becomes pattern, at his new sense of anticipation gone unfulfilled, at the high-pitched floorboards and hinges and stairs saying something he's already learned and let go of.

october 30

Last year ivy began to climb the tree: first one line, then another pointing, like fingers of frost pulling up a dark pane. I believed it grew ferociously at night. I ripped the vines from the trunk until they stretched beyond my reach. And when I hired our teenaged neighbor to do some chores, I asked him, too, to try and tear the ivy off, and he came to me saying he pulled hard but it wouldn't come down. I saw the ring of his attempt, well above the small patch I'd worked on. A few weeks later it was impossible to tell either one of us had been there.

Now all six trees in the stand of pines are covered nearly to their tops with ivy. The trunks are shirred like a rainy-day toy I made with my mother when I was young: roll a newspaper tightly into a cone and, having folded it according to pattern, cut down into it and peel back the flaps: it's a tuft of beach grass, a tassel, a tickler, a fountain of gray-and-white words to make noise with. Here are the thickened bodies of trees. And though they do not look older or frayed by the weight of their finery, it is hard to imagine them once as bare and lithe as the saplings planted curbside.

Here in our yard is the erasure rampant growth causes: the original form lost to the swaddled new face. I'd recognize the look of that anywhere.

october 31

Spots of teeth crop up in the secret chamber of his mouth; first comes a cresting of the pink gum, a tender welt, then from the new ridge, a flash of white. Then little clicks on the spoon as he works the cool metal bowl over the flare.

The light presses through the grown trees in the small field beyond my window: *field* because the grass grows tall, is tended by several boys, and foxes run through it. *Light* because it lies down in the green of morning, green of evening for nothing. Midday the light is gold cast in branches, sacks of light ripening and spilling on concrete. Morning and evening, light as sinuous as the back of a cat, the cat itself a measure of time, lazy and profligate. Time as sinuous as this light, which lies down, hides itself, gets up, grows longer, sharper, peaks, disappears into the mouth dark is.

n o v e m b e r 2

I want to make long lists of things to do, of ideas to unravel, though lists hardly help, and the words just accrete—tactile words, students', foreign, official. The words loop over and over themselves, a child's race-car set flying, the fast little machine of thought holding its place on the track by force. At the crest of a loop these days the wind dies down, Joseph cries when he's done with his nap, the formal press of momentum releases, and the thought I was holding falls and rolls to a halt. The tiny car bursts into flames and I walk away from its hissing, its ash.

Or this, another image of derailment:

An archway at the edge of a town, where huge stones make the space a cool entry in the midday heat. Beyond is a town, unguarded in its habits: the market stalls beckon, all the herbs, scarves, and pottery lemony in sun, in refracted bird colors. Past the gray of the stones, the bustle and glaze of the town open into the distance with the ease of an arm unfolding to point the way. And I'm approaching. I walk into the heart of the crowd. I'm drawn forth, but I'm also being watched. I sense the warning, *turn back,* my steps falter, the lip of my sandal catches on the uneven bricks. I'm furtive now, checking behind as I enter the long shadow of the arch thrown over the street, dark as water splashed on cobbles. From each side of the arch, hinges tune up, the two halves of a thick gate are given a push and rush together and I stop short—not fast enough to slip between—and brace for the shuddering clang of the bolt. I can see the life of the town, the freshets of color, color arrayed in tumbling ranks, going on, going on without me.

Or this:

I am as a northern god, thick-waisted with layers of skirts and a looped belt for brushes. My work for the day is heart-shaped and saw-toothed. It is the time of year for sere, dun and vermilion—the burned and burning hues—and so I settle in, staining the slight veins of leaves to show the articulated branchings within. The afternoon starts off well—taken together, the trees I've worked on move like comets in a blur of motion. I throw a brown spot, lay a mesh of red over another's face, and here, where a snapping fire passed in my mind, release an orange underglow, a flush. And then. And then, because I am a mother and the wind has called, I stop. Its high whistle slips in sharp and easy as a new key. And the part-bright tree is, for now, finished. That is, incomplete. And the unpainted leaves, the still-green ones, when the cold comes, will be holding on and on to the limbs—such dumb hope, the release not coming now, or soon even.

Or:

I am the blank, wide face of an old alarm clock balancing on two thin silver legs. A cartoon, so I can feel in big, simple ways, within the dark contours of my frame. Just before the hour hand hits its mark, the wailing starts from deep within and travels so fast I don't know what to think, I, the mechanical body of anticipation. Sketch lines for shock float like eyebrows above my head. The wide expanse of my belly, which is the face I show the world, rocks with the moment called forth. "Fetch me," says the hour now become present, urgent, extreme. What stars of pain when I fall over, off the table from such ringing. Stars circling like a crooked halo. And then I'm set upright again to tick sensibly on.

november 7

Heavy drops of rain, like ball bearings, like cable cars in tandem, run along the phone lines, then drop unexpectedly down. Rain since last evening has stained the bark of the loblollies black; it makes the garbage cans brightest where a foot kicked a dent in. And where the pine needles attach to the branch, those roots are a darker green, as if this were the place in a painting where the brush was held to the canvas longest.

Coming into the house last night, Joseph was wary and alert. There was the confusion of *wind-through-dry-leaves or rain-on-trees* all around us, the street a breathing force, drawing and expelling, pausing and blowing again. It made the street lights heave in and out of sight and patch across the tops of cars. He held both my shoulders and looked past my face into the wooded cul-de-sac. He held tightly, wanting to head out into, pushed back by the sighs rising from nowhere: another

unnamed phenomenon for him. He was looking into the
thick lung of the street, that odd animal heaving its belly,
whose body, in sleep, presents itself for full examination.
And what did my own breathlessness mean to him then, and
what could be made of my resolute walk and careful steps up
to the wet stoop, the ready key angled for the lock? And where
was I then, if not as close as a mother should be, as close as
always in the bars of shifting lights? Where was I really? And
how did it feel to be held so close to the threat I invited into
our circle, hanging back in such weather, knowing we would
be safe in minutes? What did I teach him, just then, by the
careless way I'd buttoned my jacket in the cold, slowing to
listen to the hollow night's voice, indulging the sensation
of being lost in a storm with nothing to protect me but
a child?

november 13

Yesterday I saw a cartoon—"New Fun with Dick and Jane: an
update of the 30's era classic for a more dysfunctional age." In
mock simplistic language sprinkled with jargon, Dick and Jane
and their little sister Sally try on neurosis, lit crit, and identity
politics. New captions are paired with the primer's original
drawings of the children. Dick, Jane, and Sally have lovely,
strong calves, cotton socks that sag and bunch at the ankle,
good shoes with sturdy, rounded toes. Their elbows are
shadowed with the sweaty dirt of a kid's active day, and their
hair is parted simply and combed out of their faces. They all

wear bangs. Dick wears shorts and a striped shirt. The girls'
dresses would twirl if they spun around; the sleeves are
puckered, and there's just a bit of everyday lace at their collars.
Their buffed shoes are highlighted with small, white windows
of light. When they run down the lane, past a stylized barn,
their bodies lean forward, eagerly. Sally points to a plane, and
Jane stands behind her, fist on her hip, lashes showing behind
the hillock of her cheek: she's impatient or pausing. There's
grass underfoot in tufts that seem soft under Jane's black heel.
Dick pulls a red wagon full of leafy-looking groceries (*fresh
cilantro,* the cartoon quips) and he, too, leans his whole body
into his task. Jane waves him on, her round button eyes wide,
her mouth open, a simple word forming, her eyebrows
perched high in excitement.

In another panel she receives a present from her parents; her
teeth are a solid white space in an up-curve. Her parents look
on with love, that slight tilt of the head. When their adult
bodies crouch down to meet hers, they look almost happier
than she does. There's the plane again in a puff of cloud,
propellers churning perfect half-circles.

This is the child's world as past generations read it. But
paired with this ironic text, the drawings are stark as x-rays,
denuded. The mother's and father's faces turn hard and
mechanical, their gifts appear brandished. The children's
clothes seem inauthentic, merely retro, their socks fashionably
slouchy, and the shading on their apple cheeks too precise, a
high flush that makes them look as if they've been running,
indeed for fifty years now, to keep up.

How the words make the very breath go out of them.

Their arms raised toward the dipping plane, now a salute, an act of obedience and not a simple wave in hopes the far-off pilot might have seen them.

Foolish children, foolish parents—none of this exists and nothing like it ever has, I read. *It never was. And wake up sleepers, if any remain; it will not be.* I read the ever-so-unsentimental text and feel—relegated. Miscalibrated. So *five minutes ago.* To smirk, of course, requires company, and I'm aware of the invitation extended here—but I want instead to be alone with these children. How surprising this sudden need to rescue them; what protective resolve those simple sketches have mustered in me. But then, I have seen that bare arm outstretched and waving, elbow contoured by the dark spot of a dimple. I have seen the bent back of my husband, forehead to the ground as he peers through the lowest rungs of his chair at Joseph. And the quiet way my child sits on the floor turning the dials of the stereo, as Sally is sitting on her square of floor, in front of that wildly new TV, its speakers crosshatched with burlap, the dial a little steering wheel in her plump hands. And in another frame, her finger is outstretched, pointing up to the sky—*Look!* she means, which is not "See Mother jet off to a meeting," but *Look and see what I'm seeing, it's bright, it flies, it disappears.* And yes, it does disappear, so soon: the sun takes the whole sky and whitens it fiercely so the plane dissolves, like a needle through a blanket. Or a cloud gulps it down, wings and all, every bone. Or ten planes go by; in a few years, hundreds. Then there is something newer still to look for, to search out, and the little plane is gone from sight, sooner than anyone could have imagined.

november 15

Reckless: that is, to part the body from its contingencies, to be without heed, as in: whosoever is too briefly on this earth to accumulate care and the tethering weight of consequence will surely fly off it. *Reck:* care, consider, regard . . . "Why do men now then not reck his rod?" . . . And *wreck:* that which is cast ashore by the sea; goods or cargo thrown on land from a stranded or foundered vessel. A vessel broken or ruined by being driven on rocks. An article of wreckage. The broken form of a person.

The body on the bicycle lashed with speed. The silver tongue of the slide we rode down, children out of the belly of air. Spit onto the concrete if we flew too fast, didn't catch ourselves. Legs over the sides. Dangling our arms. Going head first, face down on the cool silver, to see the reflected sky upended.

Walking along the length of seesaw until it tilted and we were pitched down and jumped over the metal handle in time. So lightly over, we carried nothing. Lightly over the speed hump, nothing but loose change in his pocket. Fast around the corner, the air warm through the open window, fast to the beach the boys were going and the girl watched them fly out of the school parking lot, saw then the light, the colors of which mean *heed,* mean *reck,* saw how over the yellow line the car went, over the wheel the boy was thrown and out the window and hard to the ground.

And nothing floated up from the sea of lights. No wreckage, and he was fathoms below, taken by the pull and salty stir of his blood. "And of his bones were coral made. Those are pearls that were his eyes." Wrecked, and reckless was the boy then, that is: without care, consideration. I mean *free*. Free to fall, without the twin weights of *if* and *then,* without the time it takes to discern, without the mechanics it takes to construct a scale of one's body, set bone against speed and measure. Decide. *Reckon*: (informal) to think or assume.

How he loved the fleet poverty of being young, no time to wait, none to spare; the poverty of the present in which his living was all clean economy of motion: nothing to save, to keep safe and *in case of.* All give, and play, this blessed immediate. The boy in the car, the speed of the car, the wind like never before (like never again) oh free, he was free, the shirt of care, its collar unbuttoned, then off entirely, the way a boy yanks it, grabbing the back first and quick over the head, the pockets upending, coins falling fast and he let them all go and they rolled, silver wheels in the sun, past the couch and under the table, behind the dark back of the dresser, everlastingly gone.

december 10

In Carlo Crivelli's *Madonna and Child,* the baby Jesus is perhaps ten months old. His halo and hers intertwine and form, above their heads (they are pressed cheek to cheek) the two round shoulders of a heart. Apples and pears, ripe as chiming bells, hang in each corner of the scene, which is all light and balanced harmonies. But best of all, the baby's tiny sandals are misstrung; the little toe of his right foot—the gorgeous, thick toes and plump heel Mary can't help touching with her long fingers—is left out of the sandal strap. In her haste. Because the child was squirming, so eager was he to get on with the day.

)))

Distinguished among mothers, the *Madonna of the Goldfinch* allows her son to hold the bird he loves in his hand. It must have been she who taught him to carry the bright bird so gently. He grasps the folds of her shawl with his free hand as she balances him in the crook of her arm, which likely is numb with his weight by now. She is looking down, noting the steep stairs as the baby peers out, over the head of the viewer, to where the birds are gathering, far off, just a handful of her soft shawl tethering him.

)))

Mary, Queen of Heaven, Ascending, is assisted by a score of bright angels—in gilt robes, in white robes, their wings cool jade, coral, and pearl, with peacock-eye designs inlaid. Her hair is a crimped flow past her breasts and the angels' hair is crimped too, but shorter. And though she is clearly on her way up from the tiny earthly castle, from dollops of lakes and thick forests below, the angels with their harps, horns, and lutes, the angels with scrolled music, singing their parts—all of them have a hand on her body, are touching her somewhere, holding fast to her heavy blue raiment, so that Mary seems stilled, held fast in midair. Caught so, she is wearing the hands of these busy attendants, accepting their efforts, their best intentions, their constant, enormous need.

)))

The visitors, Saints Stephen and Lawrence, are deep in prayer, their heads bent down. It's Florence. It's still the fifteenth century. Mary is sitting on a simple wooden throne and with her boy, receiving the guests. The baby has flung one arm around her neck and with his free hand pulls at his little rope belt. He is standing, and Mary holds one foot tightly, in her hand. He uses it as a step and soon, if the men don't finish praying, worshiping the miracle before them, the miracle will have climbed to the armrest and crawled down the dark velvet, away.

)))

Veronese's *Madonna and Child* are received by Saint Agnes, who wears thick, pinned loops of braids around her head. Mary's dark hair is simply parted and falls straight to her shoulders. She looks young, angular again; it has been perhaps six months now since the birth. Saint Agnes, with open arms and big, muscular hands, speaks to the baby, and he reaches both chubby fists out to her. And though her lovely head is illuminated by the thin gold ring of a halo, the baby sees bracelets, so close on her outstretched wrist, and stares there, inclines toward the sound, the soft, musical clinking that throws the light he emanates back and breaks it, interestingly, into a shower of irresistible sparks.

)))

In Smolensk the colors of Mary's robe are severe as winter, pooled stains of purple and black, and the baby's small gown is a deep red, etched thickly with gold, like a woodcut. He is already grown, balanced on her forearm, a tiny man painted to scale, with a receding hairline and strong, straight nose. His head is smaller than her hand, his hands and feet no bigger than her thumb. Miraculous powers are attributed to this icon, in which the child-man looks directly, piercingly out. Mary looks from behind his shoulder, not meeting the gaze of the viewer, heavy circles below her eyes, a crenellation of wrinkles in the corner of each, the flush on her cheeks the only soft gesture the painting allows amidst the blinding gold wash, gold leafing, gold frame holding the difficult pair together.

)))

The great icon painter Andrei Rublev saw Mary's eyes heavy and reddened from the start, her lips a thin line, her shoulders and head bent with the effort of sorrow. One hand is open, palm up, pleading, the other draws her dark robe closed. Behind her the clouds curve like breasts or knuckles, repeat across the sky, and are picked up again in the drape of the gown's opening. She is restrained in her private grief, a sadness known in the body, in the weight of her heavy head inclined toward—the sick child? The child hurt or unable to sleep?

The child about to leave home for the world?

But this is only one panel of an entire iconostasis. A partial view. And thus she cannot say all she knows, all she feels. Thus she can assure anyone looking to her for guidance only this: there are no words for this helplessness, no way to ease the necessity of loss.

When Joseph is gone to his babysitter, I straighten his room, take out the garbage, make taut the corners of his sheets, close the door to his dark closet.

This time last year, as his birth drew near, I'd enter the quiet room and do the same—arrange and rearrange tiny socks, blankets, underwear, ointments. We'd unwrap gifts and find them a place or store them in labeled boxes for later. But the ordering was like unpacking a stranger's suitcase, riffling the towel, robe, shirt while keeping a distance from the intimate lives of these things, soon to be touching another's skin, swiping over a face. I remembered today, too, as my body dipped and turned from the store of clean diapers on the lower shelf to wipes on the dresser, as I bent to reach the box of tissues, how impossible it was to arrange the room when we couldn't yet map our bodies' motions within it, nor could we see clearly the shapes of tasks, the functional heights or shelf space things required. So everything was neatly lined up, awaiting his arrival, as at a hotel, a good hotel, where amenities are present but still approximate: pen and paper near the phone but not comfortably in reach, or the sheets turned down not quite far enough, or too far, the slippers still wrapped in their heat-sealed packet.

)))

When we arrived home with Joseph we unwrapped him and laid him in the swinging basket, where he stayed content for hours. And then we had to think: what to do next—so we neatened the room; we hung his snowsuit in the closet next to our coats. And only then did I see that gesture, mine or Jed's, I don't remember: the snowsuit goes *here*, on this hook where it's easiest to reach, where it won't be knocked off a hanger. It was the gesture called *first time hanging the snowsuit*; my vision narrowed and I saw the movements as if through a telescope, a great distance brought unbelievably near: the closet's dimensions, the size of the snowsuit. And then I could see next summer, next fall, *arms up, sweater off*, a *child* on the floor, a child *standing*, groceries in bags then out of bags, child holding a soup can, rolling it away, as the jacket, coat, sweatshirt was hung up, or draped, or tossed, approximately, in.

)))

The first time I took him out, I needed a destination, something to hold me to the wild outside, to a sense of intention beyond his immediate needs. It had to be close, walkable, easy. So Joseph's first outing was to Val-U-Village. I walked the crammed aisles with him strapped to my chest and, like a recent immigrant to this country, was overwhelmed by the bounty. By the piles of seconds and cast-offs for sale, by the sheer mass of stuff to be cycled through. My radar off course, I saw nothing individually. I needed nothing at all. I wanted only to walk up and down the colorful aisles with my child, a weight slung against my chest, to feel the curve of his back under my hand while looking at something utterly still, while attempting something bounded and certain. I had never been dizzier, shifting my gaze from his face to T-shirts, red, buckles, organza, pillows, vests, wool, wallets. I was woozy with the task of focusing out and back, from color to form, and it still hurt to walk, to turn from his face to the offerings of the world at large. It hurt to make my eye discerning again.

december 17

I am of two minds in class this afternoon. I think: It's winter, he should put on some real shoes, for God's sake, not those sandals. I think: though he sat next to me all semester, I cannot describe even the color of his hair, was taken instead by the way he wrote furiously when seized by a compelling line, word, or moment; at how he was, so often, struck. I think: *It is starting for him, the drive, the pull* . . . but far off, you don't know this about him yet. Your son, who, here, began to work, really work: whose poems made me pause, put down my pencil in gratitude, because my own words stopped coming in the wide silence and space his cleared.

You don't yet know the writer who carries his childhood with him, the one that you and he pieced together, that he embellished; who in the course of writing his first real poems had not yet read James Wright, gone now nearly twenty years, or Elizabeth Bishop—or, really, anyone—but who stepped forth nevertheless to inhabit his own stubborn earnestness.

And though he sat next to me all semester, I did not watch his face as he spoke, knew best his voice, come from the periphery to shape a thought, that improvisational rush of right music, intellect and heart taking form, unseen, in air. In the space between us it happened and happened. *Painstaking. Easy as breathing.* This was the birth I witnessed and witnessed—this poet being born.

Stay or go, stay or go. Open the door, no, close the door, against
the cold, against the day, touch the lock, touch the knob. Wet
cars hiss: he learns *here*, he learns *gone*. Snow covers the grass,
and over dry leaves forms little tents, little depressions. Snow
paints up the west face of trees, one stroke, one layer where the
wind blew it on. It is early morning still, and the snow, fresh
and soft, pushes into the long needles of the pine. I think of
how, by the long day's end, bits of food will collect like this in
the scrub-brush, catch in the center, stick there, and have to be
worked free.

   But that is a long way off. It is still early morning and the
snow is fresh and there is time. Because the asphalt of the back
alley was warm from days of sun, the snow melted there first,
and now the alley's a dark path through the plots of grass that
grow to its edge—tight hospital corners of the neighbors'
plots, a hospital's clockwork precision laid out. It's a perfect
design on a dark cake out there, the loose sugar tapped over
the lacy cutout, oh all the cakes that came, the dishes of food,
the papery robe made sheer in the harsh light, the hospital's
white light in the baby's eyes, just minutes after he was born.
Jed's memory of the infant trying and trying to look up at that
light and blinking against its force. The sharp lines of the
glass-fronted cabinets in the delivery room, steel blue. Blue
lines of the soft cotton wraps, towels, blankets, blue stripes
along the bottom and the nurse who said *take everything home
with you*. Blue weave of a shawl, blue rickrack on towels,
a stack of them washed and folded by my mother, Jed's
mother, and the snow kept falling, falls now as we wrap our

boy up, tie his hat on, and he puts his bare hand against the pane of the front door, and the silver trash cans are blue with cold, hunkering it looks like, with sun pressing down, hurt it seems, where dents make them double over themselves in this cold.

The wooden fence, only two brown lines now, runs the perimeter of the back lot, stripes along the edge of the land, the edge of—what? Where the eye is stopped and the vision must rest, where the trees start up, where the hem of air sweeps, where the rustling passes over in shallow waves, in whispers and water breaks into rivulets on the pocked ground. The sun burns a patch through the bone white sky, and at night white comes too, ancient light down a long passage: white haze of the moon. Eggshell scattered into stars. The light of the street lamp, that skirt of white, when, as a girl, I would wake to the sound of the train across the street from my grandmother's house; it was just past the trellis of grapes our aunt grew. Past the heavy white eggplants, white peaches, white beans.

And just this afternoon, the whitest top button on the soldier's uniform: pure ivory just-so under museum light, with an X of white thread for a heart. The button was yellowed and the uniform small, and who sewed each button and then sent him off? Where the needle passed over and under and over, the loop of that motion was easy to see, as when clouds are made to part and the rays cut through. *God-rays*, how they land, cast forth so solidly, and find any of us gazing up—too simply though, and not like children, not at all like children—had I forgotten?—into the red glare.

january 4

Light out there, the color of waking to the sound of a far train, while in here a voice finds its destination: *Brrr,* he's just said, hand on the pane, as I have shown him each morning since the cold began.

Outside, the blanket of white is shrinking. A face of green is rising through it.

january 6

I keep binoculars on the windowsill so I can change four patches of white to four wet napkins fallen out of the trash; slumped rocks to brown paper bags; dangling cable, its fire enclosed, to hanging vine, its own fire waiting. Thus clarified, *barn owl* reverts to *fence post*, the wood losing, for now, its watchfulness, its hunger, its wings. And out there, near the fence, on a blue Metropolitan Museum of Art bag stuffed with newspapers, only "opol" is showing at this angle. Opal! The binoculars come down. A whole bag full, heaving and jostling, wet and leaning against the fence. In low light, a bag full of sugared violets in cream.

There's a necklace of gold around the loblolly's trunk— no, let me look: it's where the woodpecker fed, diverted the sap, and the sap hardened in beads down the north face of the tree. The vine is a mace, a spiked violence in grays, then, closer still, a tangle of nerves, each message a jolt, a wild crosscurrent.

And where the rabbit slips down into the mass of pine needles must be a gap, a proper entry, and there it is, a black depth in the brush, a depth to be filled by a body, the rabbit's. And from this distance, a motionless brown is, at first, nothing but leaves, then *a rabbit unblinking,* so close does it come through the mechanical eyes, lenses sharpening on the sack of its form, so close that the form—long ears, fur, black claws— itself becomes *rest,* that version, brief state one can wake from if startled.

january 12

The window blurs with condensation, drops held still, not floating or melting, drops unfreezing, close-knit in a huddle, like wrinkles on a turtle's leg. A ball of crepe. A crumpled letter. Cracks in. Roads in. I am watching a squirrel in the bare branches of the oak take a slip and tumble, grab hold of a limb to haul itself upright. It leaps from nothing solid at all into a net of thin branches—*twigs,* should they break, *switches,* should they be cut and wielded. Branches like stitches, crocheted and hung on the body of air. Crosshatched as a sketch in pen and ink, but one which, left out in the rain, would not dissolve away.

The squirrel leaps and figures *something will catch,* something will be there. And it is. High above, the squirrel eats black walnuts it dug, and drinks too, by pulling a dripping branch through its mouth. When it chases another squirrel down the thick trunk, they are fleet as water, pouring over the knots, a surface tremble gathering to a wave. Then it climbs again, stops, weighing thin branches. And steadied on an upper limb, the squirrel is a stone, stone-still, a poised muscle. Then suddenly, after long moments, there is—let me break it down, frame by muscle to the incrementals—an isolated, minute turn in which each limb is individually flexed and noted in concert, noted in a series of discrete, syntactical, synaptical gestures.

A squirrel studies falling until it falls well and with purpose, studies leaping and falling, rolling and falling, falling *en route* and *to get there faster,* falling and playing over limbs, over others, falling and catching itself up. Falling nearly to plunging. And by the nearest slips, I see, it learns.

)))

january 16

Refract: *"to break the course of light and turn it out of a direct line. To break the course of." To be transformed by that break, by vision reconstituted: the garbage can a* vessel *now. The raccoon's ferocity, a* mother's instinct. *The sewer a* home. Home *a known place, where walls have lumps of plaster to trace, with a finger, each morning. And gaps below doors breathe cold gusts in.*

To refract is to swerve—off the grid, the known road, and pass unhurt but wholly changed, each frequency more singular now, refined, into uncharted dark. To refract is to make many ways to that place. Where the air is thinner, where the pure air is sweeter, an intoxication, as in the story of the Magic Mountain, where

one's daily world, bounded by the body, is ever slipping away,
even as passions perform so vividly in the little theater of the
corpus.

Refracted: *"bent aside, broken down, diminished." (Obscure*
or rare: "driven back, repelled.") The moments, last winter: how
small I felt, the inconsolable moments, the crying, the exhaustion,
the walking, bouncing, the singing, rocking, walking, the crying.
Re: *"back"* + frangere: *"to break."*

All transparent bodies reflect part of the light incident
upon them. *Here is your face, child, see it in mine? Look to find*
what you feel, returned. See shades and tones herein: this, the
butter yellow of your own wariness forming, this green your joy,
and this, the reddest spot of red, let this be the long pause of
bewilderment in the face of unspeakable good fortune. Or the full
halt at the edge of a hunch: stop here. Go no further.

Refraction *occurs at the boundary between two mediums.*
At the boundary between two mediums—body to body, cheek
pressed to cheek—is a little black line into which everything falls.
Everything fills it. But no, that's not right. Black lacks hue.
Won't reflect light at all. And the boundary between us is, yet,
a warmth.

This, too, is refraction: distorting an image by viewing it
through a medium. A medium: a day, an hour, a child, fear,
hunger, awe. Inexorable growing.

Refractory: *"obstinate, unmanageable, difficult to meld."*
A refractory child. Refractory brick: elemental clay reformed and
cast and fired at high temperatures to produce a material more
durable than stone.

Yes, that which resists fire.

And will not fuse, corrode or reduce.

Such bricks were once made of the thick clay deposited by the
overflowing Tigris, the swollen Euphrates. Rivers colloidal with
clumps, shards, strands. Rained upon, churned, frothed into
motion. Bricks for dwellings of all kinds. To build with. Seen in
roofs, in steps underfoot, in the work of the Persians, and of the
Assyrians. Concealed at first by the Romans and then, uncovered
with great delight and made decorative, their internal strength
become outer: ornate, embellished, beheld.

Walking to school—such light after days of rain, beacon
after beacon urgently sent from the lighthouse every tree has
become. And once home again, great flashes fall through the
window to the wooden floor; like semaphores they redirect the
child from stairs' edge, table's corner, broken glass I rush to clear.
Fleet, broadside, the light issues forth. His hand in and out of
the puddle of sun, my own work dipped too, taken up in the
afternoon's long momentum, in its scattered deflection, in its
veer, curve, and shift.